Published in 2020

ISBN 9798643495666

The information in this book has been compiled by way of general guidance in relation to the specific subjects addressed, but is not a substitute and not to be relied on for medical, healthcare, pharmaceutical or other professional advice. Please consult your GB before changing, stopping or starting a diet. So far as the author is aware the information given is correct and up to date as at May 2020. The author disclaims, as far as the law allows, any liability arising directly or indirectly from the use, or misuse, of the information contained in this book.

Content

Intro

If you do any kind of workout you understand that what you eat defines your success and your body!

By now, you know that kitchen scales are your best friend – if not, you will find out very soon... You need to stick to your calories and macros that are in your personal meal plan as much as possible.

You also know that prepping your food can be very time-consuming, especially if you are not sure how much you should eat from certain types of food.

I know all of this, I have been through the same! I am here to help you!

With this book I am about to save you a lot of time!

When I started to do my workout and follow my meal plan, it took me a while to prepare it all correctly so I decided to create a database for myself where I entered all sorts of food and I re-searched all nutrition info for this.

I would like to share my tables with you that show calories, carbs, fat and protein for different types of food, in different amounts.

All you need to do is to look at your meal plan, match your macros with the help of this book and add it all up.

This book also contains some tips that helped me a lot, either to save time or save calories, carbs and fat.

Please be aware that this is only a guideline, based on what I usually eat. It does not include all the food that exists in the world and I did not put in any vegetarian or vegan options instead of meat. (Sorry, but I eat meat and I am not too familiar with the options vegans and vegetarians have, so I'm just sticking to what I know and use.)

Different brands might have different nutrition.

I suggest you research different brands in your country to find the most suitable product and stick to it, so you know the amount you need and you have the exact nutrition info. I left some space for you in this book where you can add your favourites.

I live in the UK, so when I refer to products, they are products available in the UK. You will need to find an alternative that is available in your country.

This book is NOT linked to any specific fitness programme.

Please pay special attention to the 'Meat', 'Rice' and 'Pasta' section!

For your own calculations: In the chapter 'How to calculate macros from the nutrition label?' I explain step by step how you can calculate your calories and macros.

I leave an empty table at the end of each chapter, so you can write there what you usually drink, eat or add your favourite brand's nutritional info.

UCW - Uncooked Weight
CW   - Cooked Weight
C   - Carb
F   - Fat
P   - Protein
tsp   - Teaspoon
tbsp - Tablespoon
US   - Unsweetened

You need your personalised meal plan to be able to use the tables in this book.

You need to know how many calories and carbs and how much fat and protein you should be consuming a day. It is different for everybody, so please make sure you choose the amount that is closest to your macros.

Yes, you do need a set of scales! It does not matter what sort of scales they are as long as they are kitchen scales. They all do one thing – measure the amount and weight of your food.

Yes, you will still need to do some maths, however the content of this book will help you massively and save you a lot of time.

The whole point of following a sustainable macro-based diet is that it's flexible. You can eat oven-baked chicken with rice and carrot for the rest of your life if you wish, but I do not think many people could and would do that. We need variety! And if you calculate your macros, you can create amazing meals all the time. You need to love what you eat, otherwise it will not be sustainable and you will not get the results you would like to see.

It would be very difficult to create a recipe book that suits everybody, as everybody needs different calorie intakes, a different macro break-down, everybody has different taste, different likes. Some people cook for 1 day, some cook for 2 or 3 days or even 5 or 6 days in advance. However, I will share some of my recipes on my **Instagram @tia.bonn**
You can also check out my website: tiabonn.com

Even if you have the recipe, you might need to adjust it. I might be able to eat 200g tomato sauce with my meal, but your macros might allow you to use only 135g, so you will need to adjust. It is better if you learn how to calculate it, so you can create your own recipes, based on what you like and you can share it with me ;)

You will need to sit down, take your time and calculate that recipe the first time, adjust if you need to adjust and write it down! You can re-use it forever and it fits your macros for sure.

This book contains a lot of food with their calories and macros, most starting from as small as 5g to 600g of weight so you do not have to look up nutrition info for each item you want to use and calculate the calories and macros, it will save you a lot of time.

Some people like using macro tracking apps and it's great if that works for you, the downsides are:
- Many of these apps allow anyone to enter anything, which means it might not be accurate.
- If the app was created let's say in the US or Europe, it will be full of American or European products but not so many from anywhere else in the world.
- You still need to enter nutrition info if you can not find it on the app.
- Many apps will have in-app purchases which means you might not be able to use all options or you can use the app only for a certain amount of time for free.

I do not put the success of my hard work in the hands of 'someone' entering the info. I research everything very carefully and to the best of my knowledge, these are the very calculations I use myself. I am also 'old-school' and like to write it down with a pen. It makes me feel good! Psychologically, if you actually write something down on a piece of paper, it is more powerful than some virtual numbers. So I am not an 'app-person' when it comes to macros.

In this book I'll give you some tips on how to save calories, carbs and fat and how to 'make up' if you are not hitting your protein target or consumed too much fat for your lunch.

I also left many empty spaces for you where you can write down YOUR favourite food. You can create your favourite breakfasts and meals and easily adjust the recipes you like.

I think if you have 3 set breakfasts, if you create 5-10 set meals for lunch/dinner from your favourites and about 3 variations for snacks, you are ready to rock! That is a very good base to start with and later, of course you can expand your very own meal-plan friendly recipe book. ☺

By the end of this book you will be able to calculate your macros easily, create your own recipes and you will have 3 breakfasts, 5-10 mains and 3 treats to get you started.

I suggest you go through the whole book first and then you can create your recipes with the help of this book and re-visit the calorie-macro tables whenever you need to.

I wish you all the best for your lifestyle change and fitness journey.

xxx

!!! MEGA-TIP !!!

This is what I do

I divided my meal plan into 3.
1 – Meal 1 – Breakfast
2 – Meal 2 – Lunch/Dinner
3 – Meal 3 – Snack

I have a set breakfast menu so I never have to calculate my macros again for my first meal, I simply pick one and this is what you will do too. I included everything you need to know to be able to put your own breakfast menu together.

I eat between midday and 17.00pm and I do intermittent fasting in-between. It means I only drink but I do not eat anything. I have my Breakfast at 12.00-12.30pm, my Lunch/Dinner at 15.30/16.00pm and my snack (If I have anything left calorie-carb-fat-wise), I will have just before 17.00pm.

If you do it this way, you can have basically anything for breakfast and for your second meal and it is very easy to see what you have left with as a snack. If you used up all your carb and fat 'allowance' for the day, then do not eat any treats on that particular day.

Treats contain a lot of carbs and fats, therefore I eat less carbs and fats during the day, so I can have my treat. On the other hand, I eat about 91% of my protein as Meal 1 and Meal 2.

This is my breakdown:

	CALORIES	CARBS	FAT	PROTEIN
MEAL 1	33%	23%	35%	40%
MEAL 2	47%	44%	46%	51%
MEAL 3	20%	33%	19%	9%

It does not mean you need to follow this, I'm just showing you a clever way to save carbs and fat for your treats and consume most of your protein before your treat. It's very easy to adjust Meal 3 if you have Meal 1 and Meal 2 planned. You might decide not to have treats but eat chips with your steak for lunch. That's why macro calculations make your meal plan easy to follow, flexible and sustainable. It's all about planning.

I like fresh food. It means I do not put vegetables, fruits or rice in the freezer. (No judgement if you do ☺) I plan my menu a week ahead to make sure I have all the ingredients I need and time planned for cooking. I cook for 2, maximum 3 days ahead. I do not like eating the same food for any longer than 3 days.

I recommend you sit down and plan your meals for the week ahead. Once you have your set breakfasts and recipes, you will know exactly what you need and how much and it will be very very easy to calculate your daily macros.

Water

Your meal plan will mention about water, so please refer to that. As a rough guideline; you should be drinking about 3-4 litres of water a day.

Tea

Tea has about **1Cal, 0C, 0F, 0P**

The best is to include some green tea as it has many positive health benefits. If you do not like the taste of green tea, I suggest you add a tea-bag of peppermint tea, it will disguise the taste a bit. If you would like to drink any other herbal tea's, black tea or fruit tea, I recommend drinking it as it is.

If you like it sweet, use **sweetener** instead of sugar. I use 'Stevia' which is the best natural sweetener in my opinion. Artificial sweeteners (saccharin, acesulfame, aspartame, neotame, and sucralose) are bad, avoid using them! Other natural low-calorie sweeteners you can try: erythritol, yacon syrup, xylitol. Sweetener however can cause bloating, so use as little as possible. Honey, coconut sugar, agave syrup and maple syrup are very high in carbs, so avoid using them.

Alcohol

Please try to avoid drinking alcohol as much as you can. I will not be preaching to you about the negative effects alcohol has on your body. From the meal plan point of view, most alcoholic beverages contain a lot of calories and carbs.

While alcohol-free beer is lower in calories than alcoholic beer, it is not completely calorie-free. Alcohol-free beers are often higher in carbs and sugar than alcoholic beer.

Beer

	CALORIES	CARBS	FAT	PROTEIN
100ML	153	13	0	2
200ML	306	26	0	3
250ML	383	32	0	4
300ML	459	38	0	4
350ML	536	44	0	5
400ML	612	51	0	6
450ML	686	57	0	7
500ML	765	63	0	8

*Include ales, lagers, porters, premium beers and stouts

Red wine

	CALORIES	CARBS	FAT	PROTEIN
100ML	85	3	0	0
150ML	128	4	0	0
200ML	170	5	0	0
250ML	213	7	0	0
300ML	255	8	0	0

White wine

	CALORIES	CARBS	FAT	PROTEIN
100ML	82	3	0	0
150ML	123	4	0	0
200ML	164	5	0	0
250ML	205	7	0	0
300ML	246	8	0	0

Vodka, Gin, Whiskey

	CALORIES	CARBS	FAT	PROTEIN
1 SHOT	116	0	0	0
2 SHOTS	231	0	0	0
3 SHOTS	347	0	0	0
4 SHOTS	462	0	0	0
5 SHOTS	578	0	0	0

*A shot is about 45ml = 45g

Rum

	CALORIES	CARBS	FAT	PROTEIN
1 SHOT	197	0	0	0
2 SHOTS	394	0	0	0
3 SHOTS	591	0	0	0
4 SHOTS	788	0	0	0
5 SHOTS	985	0	0	0

*A shot is about 45ml = 45g

Liqueurs

	CALORIES	CARBS	FAT	PROTEIN
1 SHOT	167	16	0	0
2 SHOTS	334	32	0	0
3 SHOTS	501	48	0	0
4 SHOTS	668	64	0	0
5 SHOTS	835	80	0	0

*A shot is about 45ml = 45g

Cocktails and Mixed drinks

	CALORIES	CARBS	FAT	PROTEIN
BLOODY MARY	134	9	0	1
CHOCOLATE MARTINI	341	33	8	2
COSMOPOLITAN	167	10	0	0
DAIQUIRI	244	31	0	0
GIN AND TONIC	207	15	0	0
HOT BUTTERED RUM	316	19	15	0
MAI TAI	292	24	0	0
MARGARITA	226	22	0	0
MOJITO	205	29	0	0
PINA COLADA	656	85	7	1
PORNSTAR MARTINI	224	16	0	1
RUM AND COKE	275	19	0	0
RUM AND DIET COKE	197	0	0	0
SEX ON THE BEACH	364	35	0	0
TEQUILA SUNRISE	268	42	0	0
VODKA AND COKE	194	19	0	0
VODKA AND DIET COKE	116	0	0	0
VODKA AND TONIC	189	15	0	0
WHITE RUSSIAN	574	11	30	2

*Nutrition based on standard serving size, so it is per drink, single shot

TIP: If you are making your cocktails at home, I recommend using sugar-free cocktail syrups from Jordan's Skinny Syrups - https://www.skinnymixes.com/

Soft drinks

	CALORIES	CARBS	FAT	PROTEIN
APPLE JUICE	137	34	0	0
TROPICAL JUICE	75	17	0	0
ICE TEA	57	14	0	0
PINEAPPLE JUICE	160	39	0	1
COCONUT WATER	60	12	0	2
CRANBERRY JUICE	135	33	0	0
ORANGE JUICE	135	32	0	2
COKE	112	32	0	0
DIET COKE	0	0	0	0
LEMONADE	126	35	0	0
DIET LEMONADE	0	0	0	0
FANTA	143	37	0	0
FANTA ZERO	0	0	0	0
PEPSI	128	35	0	0
PEPSI MAX	0	0	0	0

*Nutrition based on 300ml serving size

TIP: Choose the sugar-free version of soft drinks when shopping or when you are out. And drink them occasionally as 'treats'.

TIP: To make your own sugar-free drinks at home, I recommend using sugar-free syrups from Jordan's Skinny Syrups - https://www.skinnymixes.com/

Milk

I only drink unsweetened almond milk or coconut milk. I use Alpro products so my calculations below are based on that. No matter which country you live in, your best option is definitely unsweetened almond milk. It has the lowest carbs and calories amongst all milk varieties.

I do not recommend drinking cows milk for various reasons.

Your best 'guilty' meal plan friendly option - if you like coconut then of course, it's coconut milk.

You can also get unsweetened coconut milk in some countries. Unsweetened Alpro coconut milk 100ml contains 14Cal, 0C, 0F, 0P. Which means it is very similar to their unsweetened Alpro almond milk.

I will start with 50ml, because you will be using about 50ml or less for English breakfast tea, Earl Grey tea, macchiato and white americano.

You will use about 200ml for cappuccino, cereals and oat.

For latte, and protein shakes you will use about 250ml.

Alpro unsweetened almond milk
(or Alpro unsweetened coconut milk)

	CALORIES	CARBS	FAT	PROTEIN
UNSWEETENED ALMOND 50ML	7	0	0	0
UNSWEETENED ALMOND 100ML	13	0	1	0
UNSWEETENED ALMOND 150ML	20	0	1	0
UNSWEETENED	26	0	2	0

ALMOND 200ML				
UNSWEETENED	33	1	3	0
ALMOND 250ML				
UNSWEETENED	39	1	3	0
ALMOND 300ML				

Alpro coconut milk

	CALORIES	CARBS	FAT	PROTEIN
COCONUT 50ML	10	2	0	0
COCONUT 100ML	20	3	1	0
COCONUT 150ML	30	5	2	0
COCONUT 200ML	40	6	2	0
COCONUT 250ML	50	8	3	0
COCONUT 300ML	60	9	3	0

TIP: Choosing 'unsweetened' version will save you lots of carbs. It might look like a little amount, but use normal version for your coffee, for your shake and for your oat and you already consumed 180 Cal, 27C and 9F! Drink normal version occasionally as 'treat'.

Coffee

	CALORIES	CARBS	FAT	PROTEIN
SINGLE SHOT/SINGLE ESPRESSO	1	0	0	0
DOUBLE SHOT/DOUBLE ESPRESSO	2	0	0	0
BLACK AMERICANO	2	0	0	0
WHITE AMERICANO WITH 50ML UNSWEETENED ALMOND MILK	9	0	0	0
WHITE AMERICANO WITH 50ML COCONUT MILK	12	2	0	0
CAPPUCCINO WITH 200ML UNSWEETENED ALMOND MILK	28	0	2	0
CAPPUCCINO WITH 200ML COCONUT MILK	42	6	2	0
LATTE WITH 250ML UNSWEETENED ALMOND MILK	35	1	3	0
LATTE WITH 250ML COCONUT MILK	52	8	3	0

TIP: If you like your coffee sweet, you can use sweetener. You can also use sugar-free flavoured drops or skinny syrups.

16

There are many varieties out there so feel free to search the market at your leisure.

Some products that I use and recommend:
- *Flavoured drops from Myprotein – https://www.myprotein.com/*
- *Flavoured drops from Skinny Food Co. – https://theskinnyfoodco.com/*
- *Sugar-free syrups from Jordan's Skinny Syrups - https://www.skinnymixes.com/*

My drinks

Description	Weight/ amount	Calories	Carbs	Fat	Protein

Description	Weight/ amount	Calories	Carbs	Fat	Protein

Protein shake

Most protein powders have the serving size of 25g or 30g. Your meal plan will tell you how much you should be consuming. Every brand has different macros for their protein powders so the best thing to do is check yours and then calculate it. I will leave some space after my table so you can calculate and note your own calculations. To learn how to calculate your macros, please refer to the 'How to calculate macros from the nutrition label?' section in this book.

	CALORIES	CARBS	FAT	PROTEIN
25G PROTEIN WITH WATER	103	1	2	20
25G PROTEIN WITH 250 ML UNSWEETENED ALMOND MILK	136	2	5	20
25G PROTEIN WITH 250ML COCONUT MILK	153	9	5	20
30G PROTEIN WITH WATER	124	1	2	25
30G PROTEIN WITH 250G UNSWEETENED ALMOND MILK	157	2	5	25
30G PROTEIN WITH COCONUT MILK	174	9	5	25
45G PROTEIN WITH WATER	186	2	4	37
45G PROTEIN WITH 250ML UNSWEETENED ALMOND MILK	219	3	7	37
45G PROTEIN WITH COCONUT MILK	236	10	7	37

50G OF PROTEIN WITH WATER	206	2	4	41
50G OF PROTEIN WITH 250ML UNSWEETENED ALMOND MILK	239	3	7	41
50G OF PROTEIN WITH 250ML COCONUT MILK	256	10	7	41
60G OF PROTEIN WITH WATER	248	3	5	49
60G OF PROTEIN WITH 250ML UNSWEETENED ALMOND MILK	281	4	8	49
60G OF PROTEIN WITH 250ML COCONUT MILK	298	11	8	49

TIP: If you want to save some carbs, mix your protein powder with water or unsweetened almond milk.

TIP: If you add up all your macros for the day, but your protein intake is not reached, have a protein shake instead of your daily treat.

My Protein Shake

Description	Weight/ amount	Calories	Carbs	Fat	Protein

Breakfast

I will give you some breakfast options. You can use these or you can create your own at the end of this chapter. I will leave some space for you to create your 3 favourite breakfast menus.

Eggs

You can cook eggs in many different ways; boiled, fried, scrambled, poached or an omelette. Egg yolk contains the carb and fat. Egg whites only have protein.

I cook eggs in a non-stick pan and I do not use any oil. If you want to use some oil, I recommend using **extra virgin cold pressed coconut oil**, 1tsp is enough for your eggs and that contains about **39Cal, 0C, 5F, 0P** – do not forget to add this to your macros if you use some coconut oil. You can note your variation at the end of this chapter.

You can also add some vegetables to your egg, but do not forget to also add that to your calculation.

	CALORIES	CARBS	FAT	PROTEIN
1 WHOLE EGG	78	1	5	6
2 WHOLE EGGS	156	2	10	12
3 WHOLE EGGS	234	3	15	18
4 WHOLE EGGS	292	4	20	24
5 WHOLE EGGS	390	5	25	30
1 EGG WHITE	43	0	0	6
2 EGG WHTES	86	0	0	12

3 EGG WHITES	129	0	0	18
4 EGG WHITES	172	0	0	24
5 EGG WHITES	215	0	0	30
1 WHOLE EGG + 1 EGG WHITE	121	1	5	12
1 WHOLE EGG + 2 EGG WHITES	164	1	5	18
1 WHOLE EGG + 3 EGG WHITES	207	1	5	24
1 WHOLE EGG + 4 EGG WHITES	250	1	5	30
2 WHOLE EGG + 1 EGG WHITE	199	2	10	18
2 WHOLE EGG + 2 EGG WHITES	242	2	10	24
2 WHOLE EGGS + 3 EGG WHITES	285	2	10	30

TIP: Use non-stick pan if you want to save some fat.

TIP: If you have not reached your daily protein intake that is in your meal plan, eat some egg whites.

TIP: If you need to save some fat, add more egg whites and leave the yolk out of the party!

TIP: Buy some bottled egg white. It will be your new best friend!

Bottled egg white

	CALORIES	CARBS	FAT	PROTEIN
1 SERVING	22	1	0	4
2 SERVING	44	1	0	9
3 SERVING	66	2	0	14
4 SERVING	88	2	0	19
5 SERVING	110	2	0	24

*Serving size: 3tbsp

Oat – Porridge

	CALORIES	CARBS	FAT	PROTEIN
20G OAT WITH WATER	74	13	2	2
20G OAT WITH 100ML US ALMOND MILK	87	13	3	2
20G OAT WITH 100ML COCONUT MILK	94	16	3	2

30G OAT WITH WATER	110	18	2	3
30G OAT WITH 150ML US ALMOND MILK	130	18	3	3
30G OAT WITH 150ML COCONUT MILK	140	23	4	3
40G OAT WITH WATER	150	25	3	4
40G OAT WITH 200ML US ALMOND MILK	176	25	5	4
40G OAT WITH 200ML COCONUT MILK	190	25	5	4
50G OAT WITH WATER	183	31	3	6
50G OAT WITH 200ML US ALMOND MILK	209	31	5	6
50G OAT WITH 200ML COCONUT MILK	223	37	5	6

TIP: If you want to save some calories and carbs, mix your porridge with water or unsweetened almond milk.

TIP: For more variety, add some fruits or any sugar-free syrup to your porridge.

TIP: I use gluten-free instant oat and I get it from Myprotein – https://www.myprotein.com/ It has a smooth texture, I usually blend it with 200ml unsweetened almond milk (to get rid of bubble), then I pour it into a bowl and heat it in the microwave for 45seconds.

My Oat/Porridge

Description	Weight/ amount	Calories	Carbs	Fat	Protein

Cereal with milk

Research your market and find a low-fat cereal you like. Stick with it! If you stick with brands you like and enjoy, calculating your macros will be very easy. I use Honey Cheerios.

	CALORIES	CARBS	FAT	PROTEIN
20G CEREAL WITH 100ML US ALMOND MILK	94	12	3	1
20G CEREAL WITH 100ML COCONUT MILK	101	15	3	1
30G CEREAL WITH 150ML US ALMOND MILK	141	18	5	2
30G CEREAL WITH 150ML COCONUT MILK	151	23	6	2
40G CEREAL WITH 200ML US ALMOND MILK	188	25	7	3
40G CEREAL	202	31	7	3

WITH 200ML COCONUT MILK				
50G CEREAL WITH 200ML US ALMOND MILK	228	31	8	4
50G CEREAL WITH 200ML COCONUT MILK	242	37	8	4

My Cereal

Description	Weight/ amount	Calories	Carbs	Fat	Protein

Toast

Again, different types of bread have different macros so I will leave some space for you if you want to include the bread you use. I looked at different types of bread and used the highest calories, carbs, fat and average protein – this way I can pick any bread, it will fit my macros.

	CALORIES	CARBS	FAT	PROTEIN
1 SLICE OF BREAD	98	18	1	2
2 SLICES OF BREAD	196	36	2	4
3 SLICES OF BREAD	294	54	3	6
4 SLICES OF BREAD	392	72	4	8
5 SLICES OF BREAD	490	90	5	10

TIP: You can have a slice of toast with your eggs.

TIP: For low-carb pastries, pizza base, breadcrumbs, cake mixes and more, visit Lo Dough - https://lodough.co/

TIP: For low-carb high protein pasta, tortilla and bread, visit CarbZone. 1 slice of CarbZone bread contains 4C and 11P. - https://carbzone.co.uk/

TIP: You can also put low-fat sugar-free low-carb jam or spread on your bread/toast. I use jams from Skinny Food Co. – https://theskinnyfoodco.com/

Their jam per serving is 20g, must be enough for toast.
It contains: 7Cal, 5C, 0F, 0P

I use spread from Grenade Carb Killa Protein Spread -
https://www.grenade.com/uk/carb-killa-spread
Serving size is 33g, which must be enough for toast.
It contains: 176Cal, 11C, 13F, 7P

Another option I love, tastes exactly like Nutella, is Chocaholic
Hazelnut spread from Skinny Food Co. –
https://theskinnyfoodco.com/
Serving size is 5g, which is not enough for your toast,
therefore I calculated nutrition for 30g. So 30g contains:
150Cal, 17C, 12F, 0P

My Bread/Toast

Description	Weight/ amount	Calories	Carbs	Fat	Protein

HIPP and granola

I am sharing my big secret here. Haha! Yes, it is baby food! It is organic, sugar-free, gluten-free, no GM or preservatives, suitable for vegetarians and a jar is 125g which is the perfect size. I just love it! There is only a slight difference regarding to nutrition, but I used the highest calorie, carbs, fat and lowest protein content so you can pick any flavour you like. You can also use fruit puree; I'll leave some space for your favourite combinations.

	CALORIES	CARBS	FAT	PROTEIN
125G HIPP	93	21	0	1
125G HIPP WITH 20G GRANOLA	174	31	3	3
125G HIPP WITH 20G GRANOLA AND 5G COCONUT SPRINKLE	192	31	5	3
125G HIPP WITH 20G GRANOLA, 5G COCONUT SPRINKLE AND 20G BLUEBERRY	204	34	5	3
125G HIPP WITH 20G GRANOLA, 5G COCONUT SPRINKLE AND 20G STRAWBERRY	198	33	5	3
125G HIPP WITH 20G GRANOLA, 5G COCONUT SPRINKLE AND 20G RASPBERRY	203	33	5	3

My notes

Description	Weight/amount	Calories	Carbs	Fat	Protein

Protein pancake

This is my favourite, quick and easy protein pancake recipe. I am rubbish at making pancakes, but even I can make these ☺. This is your **ultimate breakfast, 3-in-1**! You will understand why. You need only 4 ingredients and I am sure you have them at home.

1 banana, 2 eggs, 35g oats and 35g protein powder.

Put everything in a blender and blend it until it is a smooth consistency and it is ready to be cooked.

It contains: **517Cal, 48C, 15F, 45P** and it means: you do not need to make a protein shake, cook eggs or porridge – **this is all-in-one**!!! You can also add more egg whites and protein powder for higher protein content.

TIP: You can add some fruits (you can find the table in 'Fruits' chapter) or you can add some sugar-free syrup. I use Zero Maple Syrup from Skinny Food Co. – https://theskinnyfoodco.com/

It is your time to put your favourite breakfast menu's together!

Based on the tables above you can now easily put your 3 favourite breakfast menu's together. You can choose it from my table or you can calculate your favourite brands nutritional values.

Here is an example menu:

Protein shake - 186Cal, 2C, 4F, 37P
Omelette – 164Cal, 1C, 5F, 18P
Cereal – 94Cal, 16C, 3F, 2P
Total – 444Cal, 19C, 16F, 57P

Make sure it fits your macros!

My favourite breakfasts

Menu 1

Description	Weight/ amount	Calories	Carbs	Fat	Protein
Total:					

Menu 2

Description	Weight/ amount	Calories	Carbs	Fat	Protein
Total:					

Menu 3

Description	Weight/ amount	Calories	Carbs	Fat	Protein
Total:					

Congratulations!!!

Now you have 3 sets of breakfast meals ☺

My notes

Description	Weight/ amount	Calories	Carbs	Fat	Protein

My notes

Description	Weight/ amount	Calories	Carbs	Fat	Protein

Lunch/Dinner

I usually have 1 meal, but you can have 2 meals by splitting it, it is up to you.

When I cook, I use my multi-cooker or air-fryer, so I do not use any oil with it.

Oil

However you might need to use some oil for some of your recipes. If that is the case, **do not forget to add this when calculating your total macros!**

	CALORIES	CARBS	FAT	PROTEIN
10ML	90	0	10	0
20ML	180	0	20	0
30ML	270	0	30	0
40ML	360	0	40	0
50ML	450	0	50	0

Use as little oil as possible.

Meat

First, you need to pick your meat. I do eat tofu as well, but only with my 'cheat meals' so I did not include it. If you use tofu, please use the empty table at the end of this section to include your own calculations. I only eat chicken breast and lean beef. But I am nice, so I created a table for fish too.

Meat is a tricky one and here is why:
Your meal plan might show the COOKED weight. Meat loses about 25% during cooking. Make sure you

understand if your meal plan contains the weight of your COOKED meat or your RAW/UNCOOKED meat, it does matter. If it shows the COOKED amount, you need to add up your daily total meat weight and add 25% = you will get the UNCOOKED weight, which you need to prep before cooking.

I calculated it all for you so all you have to do is add up the weight of your meat from your meal plan and find it in the table. It will show you all nutrition and the uncooked weight you need to buy and measure before cooking.

Cooked weight (C weight) = weight of your meat from your meal plan – total daily meat intake.

Uncooked weight (UC weight) = the amount you need to buy and measure before cooking.

TIP: I usually buy a lot of chicken and beef, cut off all the fat and then I measure it and prep portions in a bag which I then put in the freezer. So 1 bag is 1 day worth of meat.

Chicken breast

C WEIGHT	UC WEIGHT	CAL	CARBS	FAT	PROTEIN
5G	7g	9	0	0	1
10G	13g	17	0	0	2
20G	25g	33	0	0	5
30G	38g	50	0	0	8
40G	50g	66	0	1	11
50G	63g	83	0	1	14
60G	75g	99	0	1	16
70G	88g	116	0	1	19
80G	100g	132	0	1	22
90G	113g	149	0	1	25
100G	125g	165	0	2	28
125G	157g	207	0	2	35
130G	163g	215	0	2	36
135G	169g	223	0	2	37

45

140G	175g	231	0	2	39
145G	182g	240	0	2	40
150G	188g	248	0	2	42
155G	194g	256	0	3	43
160G	200g	263	0	3	44
165G	206g	273	0	3	46
170G	213g	281	0	3	47
175G	219g	289	0	3	49
180G	225g	297	0	3	50
185G	232g	306	0	3	51
190G	238g	314	0	3	53
195G	244g	322	0	3	54
200G	250g	330	0	3	56
225G	282g	372	0	4	63
250G	313g	413	0	4	70
275G	344g	454	0	4	77
300G	375g	495	0	5	84

Lean beef/steak

Choose beef with the lowest fat content you can find, it is usually written on the box.
If you buy it from a butcher like I do, cut off all the fat before weighing and cooking.

Do not eat the fat from the edges of the steak!

C WEIGHT	UC WEIGHT	CALORIES	CARBS	FAT	PROTEIN
5G	7g	7	0	1	1
10G	13g	13	0	1	2
20G	25g	26	0	2	4
30G	38g	39	0	3	7
40G	50g	52	0	3	9
50G	63g	64	0	4	12
60G	75g	77	0	5	14
70G	88g	90	0	6	17
80G	100g	103	0	7	19

90G	113g	116	0	7	22
100G	125g	128	0	8	24
125G	157g	160	0	10	30
130G	163g	165	0	11	31
135G	169g	173	0	11	33
140G	175g	179	0	12	34
145G	182g	186	0	12	35
150G	188g	192	0	12	36
155G	194g	198	0	13	37
160G	200g	205	0	13	39
165G	206g	212	0	14	40
170G	213g	218	0	14	41
175G	219g	224	0	14	42
180G	225g	231	0	15	44
185G	232g	237	0	15	45
190G	238g	244	0	16	46
195G	244g	250	0	16	47
200G	250g	256	0	16	49
225G	282g	288	0	18	55
250G	313g	320	0	20	61
275G	344g	352	0	22	67
300G	375g	384	0	24	73

Lean beef mince 5% fat

C WEIGHT	UC WEIGHT	CALORIES	CARBS	FAT	PROTEIN
5G	7g	7	0	1	1
10G	13g	13	0	1	2
20G	25g	25	0	1	4
30G	38g	38	0	2	6
40G	50g	47	0	2	8
50G	63g	62	0	3	11
60G	75g	75	0	3	13
70G	88g	87	0	4	15
80G	100g	93	0	4	17
90G	113g	112	0	5	19
100G	125g	124	0	5	22
125G	157g	155	0	7	27

130G	163g	162	0	7	28
135G	169g	168	0	7	29
140G	175g	174	0	7	30
145G	182g	180	0	8	31
150G	188g	186	0	8	33
155G	194g	193	0	8	34
160G	200g	199	0	8	35
165G	206g	205	0	9	36
170G	213g	211	0	9	37
175G	219g	217	0	9	38
180G	225g	223	0	9	39
185G	232g	230	0	10	40
190G	238g	236	0	10	41
195G	244g	242	0	10	42
200G	250g	248	0	10	44
225G	282g	279	0	12	49
250G	313g	310	0	13	55
275G	344g	341	0	14	60
300G	375g	371	0	15	66

White fish

Fish calories can be tricky because the way you prepare your fish can change the nutrition facts significantly eg. with or without skin. It also depends on what kind of fish you eat. I looked at many different varieties of fish. Because there are so many, I calculated the average of about 9 different varieties of fish. So this table shows the average white fish nutrition. I'll leave some space for you at the end of this chapter so you can add your favourite type of fish.

TIP: Calories and amount of protein is very similar in all fish. What varies is the amount of fat. My calculations are based on the average, however if you choose tuna or cod, they only have 1g of fat/100g. So you can still check macros from here for tuna and cod, but you only add 1g of fat up until 100g, 2g between 100g-200g and 3g between 200g-300g.

C WEIGHT	UC WEIGHT	CALORIES	CARBS	FAT	PROTEIN
5G	7g	6	0	0	1
10G	13g	12	0	1	2
20G	25g	23	0	1	4
30G	38g	34	0	1	6
40G	50g	43	0	1	8
50G	63g	57	0	2	10
60G	75g	68	0	2	12
70G	88g	80	0	2	14
80G	100g	91	0	2	16
90G	113g	102	0	3	18
100G	125g	113	0	3	21
125G	157g	142	0	4	26
130G	163g	147	0	4	27
135G	169g	153	0	4	28
140G	175g	159	0	4	29
145G	182g	164	0	4	30
150G	188g	170	0	4	31
155G	194g	176	0	4	32
160G	200g	181	0	4	33
165G	206g	187	0	5	34
170G	213g	193	0	5	35
175G	219g	198	0	5	36
180G	225g	204	0	5	37
185G	232g	210	0	5	38
190G	238g	215	0	5	39
195G	244g	221	0	5	40
200G	250g	226	0	5	42
225G	282g	255	0	6	47
250G	313g	283	0	7	52
275G	344g	311	0	7	57
300G	375g	339	0	8	63

49

My notes

Description	Weight/ amount	Calories	Carbs	Fat	Protein

Vegetables

Next - if you are about to cook – you need to pick your vegetables or ingredients of your salad. With salad you can get very creative and add some yoghurt or nuts, olives or avocado. If you do this, just make sure you add the macros up correctly.

You can also get some mixed vegetables to oven bake or cook in a wok. I included these too in the tables below.

If your meal plan shows salad and vegetables separately, you can swap the salad for veggies or the veggies for salad. As long as it stays within your given calorie and carb amount (be as close as you possibly can), it's okay. Your body does not know if it is getting carbs from red pepper and tomato or green beans and corn.

I included tomato paste/puree under tomato – it does not have the same nutrition.

I start with small amounts and go up gradually, it means you can easily mix and match your veggies.

I'll start with onion and garlic as we use those the most for cooking and I will continue with high calorie-carb veggies.

Onion

	CALORIES	CARBS	FAT	PROTEIN
5G	2	0	0	0
10G	4	1	0	0
15G	6	1	0	0
20G	8	2	0	0
25G	10	3	0	0
30G	12	3	0	0
35G	14	3	0	0
40G	15	4	0	0
45G	18	4	0	0
50G	20	4	0	0
55G	22	5	0	0
60G	24	5	0	0
65G	26	6	0	0
70G	28	6	0	0
75G	30	7	0	1
80G	32	7	0	1
85G	34	8	0	1
90G	36	8	0	1
95G	38	9	0	1
100G	40	9	0	1
125G	50	12	0	1
150G	60	14	0	2
175G	70	16	0	2
200G	80	18	0	2
225G	90	21	0	3
250G	100	23	0	3
275G	110	25	0	3
300G	120	27	0	3

Garlic

	CALORIES	CARB	FAT	PROTEIN
1 CLOVE	4	1	0	0
2 CLOVES	8	2	0	0
3 CLOVES	12	3	0	0
4 CLOVES	16	4	0	0
5 CLOVES	20	5	0	0

Chickpeas

	CALORIES	CARBS	FAT	PROTEIN
5G	6	1	0	0
10G	12	2	0	0
15G	18	3	0	1
20G	23	3	1	1
25G	29	4	1	1
30G	35	5	1	2
35G	41	5	1	2
40G	46	6	1	2
45G	52	7	1	3
50G	58	7	2	3
55G	64	8	2	3
60G	69	9	2	4
65G	75	9	2	4
70G	81	10	2	4
75G	87	11	2	5
80G	92	11	2	5
85G	98	12	2	5
90G	104	13	2	6
95G	110	13	3	6
100G	115	14	3	6
125G	144	17	3	8
150G	173	21	4	10
175G	202	24	4	11
200G	230	28	5	13
225G	259	31	5	15

250G	288	34	6	16
275G	317	38	6	18
300G	345	41	7	20

Peas

	CALORIES	CARBS	FAT	PROTEIN
5G	5	1	0	0
10G	9	2	0	0
15G	13	3	0	0
20G	17	3	0	1
25G	21	4	0	1
30G	25	5	0	1
35G	29	5	0	1
40G	33	6	0	2
45G	37	7	0	2
50G	41	7	0	2
55G	45	8	0	2
60G	49	9	0	3
65G	53	10	0	3
70G	57	10	0	3
75G	61	11	0	3
80G	65	11	0	4
85G	69	12	0	4
90G	73	13	0	4
95G	77	14	0	4
100G	81	14	0	5
125G	102	18	0	6
150G	122	21	0	7
175G	142	25	0	8
200G	162	28	0	10
225G	183	32	0	11
250G	203	35	0	12
275G	223	39	0	13
300G	243	42	0	15

Beans

	CALORIES	CARBS	FAT	PROTEIN
5G	7	2	0	0
10G	14	3	0	0
15G	20	4	0	1
20G	27	5	0	1
25G	33	6	0	2
30G	40	8	0	2
35G	47	9	0	3
40G	53	10	0	3
45G	60	11	0	4
50G	66	12	0	4
55G	73	13	0	4
60G	80	14	0	5
65G	86	16	0	5
70G	93	17	0	6
75G	99	18	0	6
80G	106	20	0	6
85G	113	21	0	7
90G	119	22	0	7
95G	126	23	0	8
100G	132	24	1	8
125G	165	30	1	10
150G	198	36	1	13
175G	231	42	1	15
200G	264	48	1	17
225G	297	54	2	19
250G	330	60	2	21
275G	363	66	2	23
300G	396	72	2	25

Lentils

	CALORIES	CARBS	FAT	PROTEIN
5G	6	1	0	0
10G	12	2	0	0
15G	18	3	0	1
20G	24	4	0	1
25G	29	5	0	2
30G	35	6	0	2
35G	41	7	0	3
40G	47	8	0	3
45G	53	9	0	4
50G	58	10	0	4
55G	64	11	0	4
60G	70	12	0	5
65G	76	13	0	5
70G	82	14	0	6
75G	87	15	0	6
80G	93	16	0	7
85G	99	17	0	7
90G	105	18	0	8
95G	111	19	0	8
100G	116	20	0	9
125G	145	25	0	11
150G	174	30	0	13
175G	203	35	0	15
200G	232	40	0	18
225G	261	45	0	20
250G	290	50	0	22
275G	319	55	0	24
300G	348	60	0	27

Red lentil

	CALORIES	CARBS	FAT	PROTEIN
5G	5	0	0	0
10G	10	2	0	0
15G	15	2	0	1
20G	20	3	0	1
25G	24	3	0	1
30G	29	4	0	2
35G	34	5	0	2
40G	39	5	0	2
45G	43	6	0	3
50G	48	6	0	3
55G	53	7	0	4
60G	58	8	0	4
65G	63	8	0	4
70G	68	9	0	5
75G	72	9	0	5
80G	77	10	0	6
85G	82	11	0	6
90G	87	11	0	6
95G	92	12	0	6
100G	96	12	0	7
125G	120	15	1	9
150G	144	18	1	10
175G	168	21	1	12
200G	192	24	1	14
225G	217	26	1	16
250G	240	30	2	18
275G	264	33	2	20
300G	288	36	2	21

Parsnip

	CALORIES	CARBS	FAT	PROTEIN
5G	4	1	0	0
10G	7	2	0	0
15G	10	2	0	0
20G	13	3	0	0
25G	17	4	0	0
30G	20	4	0	0
35G	24	5	0	0
40G	27	5	0	0
45G	30	6	0	0
50G	33	7	0	0
55G	34	7	0	0
60G	40	8	0	1
65G	43	9	0	1
70G	47	9	0	1
75G	50	10	0	1
80G	53	10	0	1
85G	57	11	0	1
90G	60	12	0	1
95G	63	12	1	1
100G	66	13	1	1
125G	83	16	1	2
150G	99	19	2	2
175G	116	22	2	3
200G	132	25	3	3
225G	149	29	3	4
250G	165	32	3	4
275G	182	35	4	4
300G	198	38	4	5

Corn

	CALORIES	CARBS	FAT	PROTEIN
5G	3	0	0	0
10G	6	0	0	0
15G	9	1	0	0
20G	12	1	0	0
25G	15	2	0	0
30G	18	2	0	0
35G	21	2	0	0
40G	24	3	0	0
45G	27	3	0	0
50G – HALF A COB	30	3	0	1
55G	33	4	0	1
60G	36	4	0	1
65G	39	4	0	1
70G	42	5	0	1
75G	45	5	0	1
80G	48	5	0	1
85G	51	6	0	1
90G	54	6	0	1
95G	57	6	0	1
100G – 1 COB	60	6	0	2
125G	75	8	0	2
150G	90	9	0	3
175G	105	11	0	3
200G – 2 COBS	120	12	0	4
225G	135	14	0	4
250G	150	15	0	5
275G	165	17	0	5
300G – 3 COBS	180	18	0	6

Butternut squash

	CALORIES	CARBS	FAT	PROTEIN
5G	3	1	0	0
10G	5	2	0	0
15G	7	2	0	0
20G	9	3	0	0
25G	12	3	0	0
30G	14	4	0	0
35G	16	5	0	0
40G	18	5	0	0
45G	21	6	0	0
50G	23	6	0	0
55G	25	7	0	0
60G	27	8	0	0
65G	30	8	0	0
70G	32	9	0	0
75G	34	9	0	0
80G	36	10	0	0
85G	39	11	0	0
90G	41	11	0	0
95G	43	12	0	0
100G	54	12	0	1
125G	57	15	0	1
150G	68	18	0	1
175G	79	21	0	1
200G	90	24	0	2
225G	102	27	0	2
250G	113	30	0	2
275G	124	33	0	2
300G	135	36	0	3

Tenderstem broccoli

	CALORIES	CARBS	FAT	PROTEIN
5G	3	0	0	0
10G	4	0	0	0
15G	7	0	0	0
20G	9	0	0	0
25G	11	1	0	1
30G	13	1	0	1
35G	16	1	0	1
40G	18	1	0	1
45G	20	2	0	1
50G	22	2	0	1
55G	24	2	0	2
60G	26	2	0	2
65G	28	2	0	2
70G	31	2	0	3
75G	33	3	0	3
80G	35	3	0	3
85G	37	3	0	3
90G	39	3	0	3
95G	41	3	0	4
100G	43	4	0	4
125G	54	4	0	5
150G	65	5	0	6
175G	76	6	0	7
200G	86	7	0	8
225G	97	8	0	9
250G	108	8	0	10
275G	119	9	0	11
300G	129	10	0	12

Babycorn

	CALORIES	CARBS	FAT	PROTEIN
5G	3	0	0	0
10G	5	1	0	0
15G	7	1	0	0
20G	9	2	0	0
25G	11	2	0	0
30G	13	2	0	0
35G	15	3	0	0
40G	17	3	0	0
45G	19	3	0	0
50G	21	4	0	1
55G	24	4	0	1
60G	26	4	0	1
65G	28	5	0	1
70G	30	5	0	1
75G	32	5	0	1
80G	34	6	0	1
85G	36	6	0	1
90G	38	6	0	1
95G	40	7	0	1
100G	42	7	0	2
125G	53	8	0	2
150G	63	10	0	3
175G	74	12	0	3
200G	84	13	0	4
225G	95	15	0	4
250G	105	16	0	5
275G	116	18	0	5
300G	126	20	0	6

Red cabbage

	CALORIES	CARBS	FAT	PROTEIN
5G	2	1	0	0
10G	4	1	0	0
15G	5	2	0	0
20G	7	2	0	0
25G	8	2	0	0
30G	10	3	0	0
35G	11	3	0	0
40G	13	3	0	0
45G	14	4	0	0
50G	16	4	0	0
55G	18	4	0	0
60G	19	5	0	0
65G	21	5	0	0
70G	22	5	0	0
75G	24	6	0	0
80G	25	6	0	0
85G	27	6	0	0
90G	28	7	0	0
95G	30	7	0	0
100G	31	7	0	1
125G	39	9	0	1
150G	47	11	0	1
175G	55	13	0	1
200G	62	14	0	2
225G	70	16	0	2
250G	78	18	0	2
275G	86	20	0	2
300G	93	21	0	3

Sugar snap peas

	CALORIES	CARBS	FAT	PROTEIN
5G	2	1	0	1
10G	4	1	0	1
15G	6	1	0	1
20G	7	1	0	1
25G	9	2	0	1
30G	11	2	0	1
35G	12	2	0	1
40G	14	2	0	1
45G	16	3	0	1
50G	17	3	0	1
55G	19	3	0	1
60G	21	3	0	1
65G	23	4	0	2
70G	24	4	0	2
75G	26	4	0	2
80G	28	4	0	2
85G	29	5	0	2
90G	31	5	0	2
95G	33	5	0	3
100G	34	5	0	3
125G	43	7	0	4
150G	51	8	0	4
175G	60	9	0	5
200G	68	10	0	6
225G	77	12	0	7
250G	85	13	0	8
275G	94	14	0	9
300G	102	15	0	10

Green beans

	CALORIES	CARBS	FAT	PROTEIN
5G	2	1	0	0
10G	4	1	0	0
15G	6	2	0	0
20G	7	2	0	0
25G	9	2	0	0
30G	11	3	0	0
35G	13	3	0	0
40G	14	4	0	0
45G	16	4	0	0
50G	18	4	0	0
55G	20	5	0	1
60G	21	5	0	1
65G	23	6	0	1
70G	25	6	0	1
75G	27	6	0	1
80G	28	7	0	1
85G	30	7	0	1
90G	32	8	0	1
95G	34	8	0	1
100G	35	8	0	1
125G	44	10	1	2
150G	53	12	1	2
175G	62	14	1	3
200G	70	16	1	3
225G	79	18	1	4
250G	88	20	1	4
275G	97	22	1	5
300G	105	24	1	5

Mixed salad

	CALORIES	CARBS	FAT	PROTEIN
5G	3	1	0	0
10G	5	1	0	0
50G	26	2	1	0
75G	39	3	2	0
100G	54	4	2	1
125G	64	5	3	1
150G	77	6	3	1
175G	90	7	4	2
200G	102	8	4	2
225G	115	9	5	2
250G	128	10	5	3
275G	141	11	6	3
300G	153	12	6	3

Mixed oven-bake vegetables

	CALORIES	CARBS	FAT	PROTEIN
5G	3	1	0	0
10G	6	1	0	0
50G	30	3	1	0
75G	45	5	2	1
100G	60	6	2	1
125G	75	8	3	2
150G	90	9	3	2
175G	105	11	4	2
200G	120	12	4	3
225G	135	14	5	3
250G	150	15	5	4
275G	165	17	6	4
300G	180	18	6	4

Mixed wok vegetables

	CALORIES	CARBS	FAT	PROTEIN
5G	4	1	0	0
10G	8	2	1	0
50G	34	6	2	0
75G	51	9	3	1
100G	67	12	3	1
125G	84	15	4	1
150G	101	18	5	2
175G	118	21	6	2
200G	134	24	6	3
225G	151	27	7	3
250G	168	30	8	3
275G	185	33	9	4
300G	201	36	9	4

Romano peppers

	CALORIES	CARBS	FAT	PROTEIN
5G	2	1	0	0
10G	4	1	0	0
15G	6	1	0	0
20G	8	2	0	0
25G	9	2	0	0
30G	11	2	0	0
35G	13	3	0	0
40G	15	3	0	0
45G	17	3	0	0
50G	18	3	0	0
55G	20	4	0	0
60G	22	4	0	0
65G	24	4	0	0
70G	26	5	0	0
75G	27	5	0	0
80G	29	5	0	0
85G	31	6	0	0

90G	33	6	0	0
95G	35	6	0	0
100G	36	6	0	1
125G	45	8	0	1
150G	54	9	0	1
175G	63	11	0	1
200G	72	12	0	2
225G	81	14	0	2
250G	90	15	0	2
275G	99	17	0	2
300G	108	18	0	3

Broccoli

	CALORIES	CARBS	FAT	PROTEIN
5G	2	1	0	0
10G	4	1	0	0
15G	5	1	0	0
20G	7	2	0	0
25G	8	2	0	0
30G	10	2	0	0
35G	12	3	0	0
40G	13	3	0	0
45G	14	3	0	1
50G	16	3	0	1
55G	18	4	0	1
60G	19	4	0	1
65G	21	4	0	1
70G	22	5	0	1
75G	24	5	0	1
80G	25	5	0	1
85G	27	6	0	2
90G	28	6	0	2
95G	30	6	0	2
100G	31	6	0	2
125G	39	8	0	3
150G	47	9	0	3

	CALORIES	CARBS	FAT	PROTEIN
175G	55	11	0	4
200G	62	12	0	5
225G	70	14	0	5
250G	78	15	0	6
275G	86	17	0	6
300G	93	18	0	7

Parsley

	CALORIES	CARBS	FAT	PROTEIN
1 TBSP - 4G	2	1	0	0
2 TBSP - 8G	3	1	0	0
3 TBSP - 12G	5	1	0	0
4 TBSP - 16G	6	1	0	0
5 TBSP - 20G	8	2	0	0
6 TBSP - 24G	9	2	0	0
7 TBSP - 28G	11	2	0	0
8 TBSP - 32G	12	2	0	0
9 TBSP - 36G	13	3	0	0
10 TBSP - 40G	15	3	0	0

*1tbsp of fresh parsley is about 4g

Coriander

	CALORIES	CARBS	FAT	PROTEIN
1 TBSP - 4G	1	1	0	0
2 TBSP - 8G	2	1	0	0
3 TBSP - 12G	3	1	0	0
4 TBSP - 16G	4	1	0	0
5 TBSP - 20G	5	1	0	0
6 TBSP - 24G	6	1	0	0
7 TBSP - 28G	7	1	0	0
8 TBSP - 32G	8	2	0	0
9 TBSP - 36G	9	2	0	0
10 TBSP - 40G	10	2	0	0

*1tbsp of fresh coriander is about 4g

Carrot

	CALORIES	CARBS	FAT	PROTEIN
5G	2	1	0	0
10G	4	1	0	0
15G	6	2	0	0
20G	7	2	0	0
25G	9	3	0	0
30G	11	3	0	0
35G	13	3	0	0
40G	14	4	0	0
45G	16	4	0	0

50G	18	5	0	0
55G	20	5	0	0
60G	21	5	0	0
65G	23	6	0	0
70G	25	6	0	0
75G	27	7	0	0
80G	28	7	0	0
85G	30	7	0	0
90G	32	8	0	0
95G	34	8	0	0
100G	35	9	0	0
125G	44	11	0	1
150G	53	13	0	1
175G	62	15	0	1
200G	70	17	0	1
225G	79	19	0	1
250G	88	21	0	2
275G	97	23	1	2
300G	105	25	1	2

Mixed baby leaves

	CALORIES	CARBS	FAT	PROTEIN
50G	13	2	0	0
100G	26	3	1	1
150G	39	4	2	2
200G	52	6	2	3
250G	65	7	2	4
300G	78	8	3	4
350G	91	10	3	5
400G	104	11	4	6
450G	117	12	4	7
500G	130	13	4	8

Rocket

	CALORIES	CARBS	FAT	PROTEIN
50G	13	2	1	1
100G	25	4	1	2
150G	38	6	2	3
200G	50	8	2	5
250G	63	10	2	6
300G	75	12	3	7
350G	88	13	3	9
400G	100	15	3	10
450G	113	17	4	11
500G	125	19	4	13

Spinach

	CALORIES	CARBS	FAT	PROTEIN
50G	12	2	1	1
100G	23	4	1	3
150G	35	6	1	4
200G	46	8	1	6
250G	58	10	1	7
300G	69	12	1	9
350G	81	14	2	10
400G	92	16	2	12
450G	104	18	2	13
500G	115	19	2	15

Tomato

	CALORIES	CARBS	FAT	PROTEIN
5G	2	1	0	0
10G	3	1	0	0
15G	4	1	0	0
20G	6	1	0	0
25G	7	1	0	0

	CALORIES	CARBS	FAT	PROTEIN
30G	8	2	0	0
35G	10	2	0	0
40G	11	2	0	0
45G	12	2	0	0
50G	13	2	0	0
55G	15	3	0	0
60G	16	3	0	0
65G	17	3	0	0
70G	19	3	0	0
75G	20	3	0	0
80G	21	4	0	0
85G	23	4	0	0
90G	24	4	0	0
95G	25	4	0	1
100G	26	4	0	1
125G	33	5	1	1
150G	39	6	1	1
175G	46	7	1	1
200G	52	8	1	2
225G	59	9	2	2
250G	65	10	2	2
275G	72	11	2	3
300G	78	12	2	3

Tomato puree (concentrated)

	CALORIES	CARBS	FAT	PROTEIN
20G	19	4	0	0
40G	38	7	0	1
60G	57	11	0	2
80G	76	14	0	3
100G	97	18	0	4

*Serving size is 20g

73

Spring onion

	CALORIES	CARBS	FAT	PROTEIN
5G	2	1	0	0
10G	3	1	0	0
15G	4	1	0	0
20G	5	1	0	0
25G	6	1	0	0
30G	8	1	0	0
35G	9	2	0	0
40G	10	2	0	0
45G	11	2	0	0
50G	12	2	0	1
55G	14	2	0	1
60G	15	2	0	1
65G	16	2	0	1
70G	17	2	0	1
75G	18	3	0	1
80G	20	3	0	1
85G	21	3	0	1
90G	22	3	0	1
95G	23	3	0	1
100G	24	3	0	2

Bell pepper

	CALORIES	CARBS	FAT	PROTEIN
5G	2	1	0	0
10G	3	1	0	0
15G	5	2	0	0
20G	6	2	0	0
25G	7	2	0	0
30G	9	3	0	0
35G	10	3	0	0
40G	12	3	0	0
45G	13	3	0	0
50G	14	4	0	0

	CALORIES	CARBS	FAT	PROTEIN
55G	16	4	0	0
60G	17	5	0	0
65G	19	5	0	0
70G	20	5	0	0
75G	21	6	0	0
80G	23	6	0	0
85G	24	6	0	0
90G	26	7	0	0
95G	27	7	0	0
100G	28	7	0	0
125G	35	9	0	1
150G	42	10	0	1
175G	49	12	0	1
200G	56	14	0	1
225G	63	16	0	2
250G	70	17	0	2
275G	77	18	0	2
300G	84	21	0	2

Bean sprouts

	CALORIES	CARBS	FAT	PROTEIN
5G	2	1	0	0
10G	3	1	0	0
20G	6	1	0	0
25G	7	1	0	0
30G	9	1	0	0
40G	11	2	0	0
50G	14	2	0	1
60G	17	2	0	1
70G	19	3	0	1
75G	21	3	0	1
80G	22	3	0	1
90G	25	3	0	2
100G	27	4	0	2
125G	34	4	0	2
150G	41	5	0	3

	CALORIES	CARBS	FAT	PROTEIN
175G	48	6	1	4
200G	54	7	2	4
225G	61	8	2	5
250G	68	8	2	5
275G	75	9	2	6
300G	81	10	2	6

Mushroom

	CALORIES	CARBS	FAT	PROTEIN
5G	2	1	0	0
10G	3	1	0	0
20G	6	2	0	0
25G	7	2	0	0
30G	9	2	0	0
40G	12	3	0	0
50G	14	3	0	1
60G	17	4	0	1
70G	20	4	0	1
75G	21	4	0	1
80G	23	5	0	1
90G	26	5	0	1
100G	28	6	0	2
125G	35	7	0	2
150G	42	8	0	3
175G	49	10	0	3
200G	56	11	1	4
225G	63	12	2	4
250G	70	14	2	5
275G	77	15	2	6
300G	84	16	2	6

White cabbage

	CALORIES	CARBS	FAT	PROTEIN
5G	2	1	0	0
10G	3	1	0	0
15G	4	1	0	0
20G	5	2	0	0
25G	6	2	0	0
30G	7	2	0	0
35G	8	2	0	0
40G	9	2	0	0
45G	10	3	0	0
50G	11	3	0	0
55G	12	3	0	0
60G	13	4	0	0
65G	14	4	0	0
70G	16	4	0	0
75G	17	4	0	0
80G	18	5	0	0
85G	19	5	0	0
90G	20	5	0	0
95G	21	5	0	1
100G	22	6	0	1
125G	28	7	0	1
150G	33	8	0	1
175G	39	10	0	1
200G	44	11	0	2
225G	50	12	0	2
250G	55	13	0	2
275G	61	15	0	3
300G	66	16	0	3

Aubergine

	CALORIES	CARBS	FAT	PROTEIN
5G	1	0	0	0
10G	2	1	0	0
20G	4	1	0	0
25G	5	1	0	0
30G	6	1	0	0
40G	8	1	0	0
50G	10	2	0	0
60G	12	2	0	0
70G	14	2	0	0
75G	15	2	0	0
80G	16	2	0	0
90G	18	2	0	0
100G	20	3	0	0
125G	25	3	1	1
150G	30	3	1	1
175G	35	5	1	1
200G	40	5	1	1
225G	45	5	1	2
250G	50	6	1	2
275G	55	7	1	2
300G	60	6	1	2
350G	70	8	2	3
400G	80	9	2	3
450G	90	10	2	4
500G	100	11	2	4

Cauliflower

	CALORIES	CARBS	FAT	PROTEIN
5G	1	0	0	0
10G	2	0	0	0
20G	5	1	0	0
25G	6	1	0	0
30G	7	2	0	0
40G	10	2	0	0
50G	12	3	0	0
60G	14	3	0	1
70G	17	3	0	1
75G	18	3	0	1
80G	19	4	0	1
90G	21	4	0	1
100G	23	5	0	1
125G	29	6	0	2
150G	35	7	0	2
175G	41	8	0	3
200G	46	9	1	3
225G	52	10	1	4
250G	58	11	2	4
275G	64	12	2	4
300G	69	13	2	5
350G	81	15	2	6
400G	92	17	2	7
450G	104	19	3	8
500G	115	21	3	9

Asparagus

	CALORIES	CARBS	FAT	PROTEIN
5G	2	0	0	0
10G	3	1	0	0
20G	5	1	0	0
25G	6	1	0	0
30G	7	2	0	0
40G	9	2	0	0
50G	11	3	0	1
60G	14	3	0	1
70G	16	3	0	1
75G	17	4	0	1
80G	18	4	0	1
90G	20	4	0	2
100G	22	5	0	2
125G	28	6	0	3
150G	33	7	0	3
175G	39	8	0	4
200G	44	9	0	4
225G	50	10	0	5
250G	55	11	0	6
275G	61	12	0	6
300G	66	13	0	7
350G	77	15	0	8
400G	88	17	0	9
450G	99	19	0	10
500G	110	21	1	12

Bamboo shoots

	CALORIES	CARBS	FAT	PROTEIN
5G	2	0	0	0
10G	3	1	0	0
15G	5	1	0	0
20G	6	1	0	0
25G	7	2	0	0
30G	9	2	0	0
35G	10	2	0	0
40G	11	2	0	1
45G	13	3	0	1
50G	14	3	0	1
55G	15	3	0	1
60G	17	4	0	1
65G	18	4	0	1
70G	19	4	0	1
75G	21	4	0	1
80G	22	5	0	2
85G	23	5	0	2
90G	25	5	0	2
95G	26	5	0	2
100G	27	6	0	2

Courgette

	CALORIES	CARBS	FAT	PROTEIN
5G	1	0	0	0
10G	2	1	0	0
20G	3	1	0	0
25G	4	1	0	0
30G	5	1	0	0
40G	6	1	0	0
50G	8	2	0	0
60G	9	2	0	0
70G	10	2	0	0
75G	11	2	0	0

80G	12	3	0	0
90G	14	3	0	0
100G	15	3	0	1
125G	19	4	0	1
150G	23	4	0	1
175G	27	5	0	1
200G	30	6	0	2
225G	34	6	0	2
250G	38	7	0	2
275G	42	8	1	3
300G	45	9	1	3
350G	53	10	1	3
400G	60	11	2	4
450G	68	13	2	4
500G	75	14	2	5

Jalapeno

	CALORIES	CARBS	FAT	PROTEIN
5G	1	0	0	0
10G	1	1	0	0
15G	2	1	0	0
20G	3	1	0	0
25G	4	1	0	0
30G	5	2	0	0
35G	6	2	0	0
40G	7	2	0	0
45G	8	2	0	0
50G	9	2	0	0
55G	10	2	0	0
60G	11	3	0	1
65G	12	3	0	1
70G	13	3	0	1
75G	14	3	0	1
80G	15	3	0	1
85G	16	4	0	1
90G	17	4	0	1

	CALORIES	CARBS	FAT	PROTEIN
95G	18	4	0	1
100G	19	4	0	1

Cucumber

	CALORIES	CARBS	FAT	PROTEIN
5G	1	0	0	0
10G	2	0	0	0
20G	3	1	0	0
25G	4	1	0	0
30G	5	1	0	0
40G	6	2	0	0
50G	8	2	0	0
60G	9	3	0	0
70G	10	3	0	0
75G	10	3	0	0
80G	12	3	0	0
90G	14	4	0	0
100G	15	4	0	0
125G	19	5	0	0
150G	23	6	0	1
175G	27	7	0	1
200G	30	8	0	1
225G	34	9	0	1
250G	38	9	0	1
275G	42	10	0	1
300G	45	11	0	2
350G	53	13	0	2
400G	60	15	0	2
450G	68	17	0	3
500G	75	18	0	3

Lettuce

	CALORIES	CARBS	FAT	PROTEIN
5G	1	0	0	0
10G	2	0	0	0
20G	3	1	0	0
25G	4	1	0	0
30G	5	1	0	0
40G	6	2	0	0
50G	7	2	0	0
60G	9	2	0	0
70G	10	3	0	0
75G	11	3	0	0
80G	12	3	0	0
90G	13	3	0	0
100G	14	3	0	0
125G	18	4	0	1
150G	21	5	0	1
175G	25	6	0	1
200G	28	6	0	1
225G	32	7	0	2
250G	35	8	0	2
275G	39	9	0	2
300G	42	9	0	2
350G	49	11	0	3
400G	56	12	0	3
450G	63	14	0	4
500G	70	15	0	4

Pick your side

Rice

Rice and pasta are tricky too. They take up a lot of water. Make sure you understand whether your meal plan show the COOKED or the UNCOOKED amount you need to consume. If it shows the uncooked amount, it's easy, if it shows the COOKED amount, then you need to know that the **weight of rice multiplies by 3 for the time it's cooked**. For example: if your meal plan says you need to eat 50g rice (cooked), it means you need to weigh 17g of uncooked rice before cooking. Don't panic, it's all calculated for you below.

(C weight = Cooked weight; UC weight = Uncooked weight)

White Basmati Rice/White rice

C WEIGHT	UC WEIGHT	CALORIES	CARBS	FAT	PROTEIN
5G	1.7g	6	2	0	0
10G	3g	11	3	0	0
20G	7g	25	6	0	0
25G	8g	29	7	0	0
30G	10g	36	9	0	0
40G	13g	46	11	0	1
50G	17g	60	15	0	1
60G	20g	71	17	0	1
70G	23g	81	20	0	1
75G	25g	88	21	0	2
80G	27g	95	23	0	2
90G	30g	106	26	0	2
100G	33g	116	28	0	2
110G	37g	130	31	0	2
120G	40g	141	34	0	3
130G	43g	151	36	0	3
140G	47g	165	40	0	3
150G	50g	176	42	0	4

160G	53g	187	45	0	4
170G	57g	200	48	0	4
180G	60g	211	51	0	4
190G	63g	222	53	0	5
200G	67g	236	56	0	5
210G	70g	246	59	0	5
220G	73g	257	62	0	5
230G	77g	271	65	0	6
240G	80g	281	67	0	6
250G	83g	292	70	0	6
260G	87g	306	73	0	7
270G	90g	316	76	0	7
280G	93g	327	78	0	7
290G	97g	341	82	0	7
300G	100g	351	84	0	8

Brown Basmati Rice

C WEIGHT	UC WEIGHT	CALORIES	CARBS	FAT	PROTEIN
5G	1.7g	6	1	0	0
10G	3g	11	3	0	0
20G	7g	25	6	0	0
25G	8g	29	7	0	0
30G	10g	36	8	0	0
40G	13g	47	11	0	1
50G	17g	61	14	0	1
60G	20g	71	16	1	1
70G	23g	82	18	1	1
75G	25g	89	20	1	2
80G	27g	96	22	1	2
90G	30g	107	24	1	2
100G	33g	118	26	1	2
110G	37g	132	29	2	3
120G	40g	142	32	2	3
130G	43g	153	34	2	3
140G	47g	167	37	2	4
150G	50g	178	39	2	4
160G	53g	189	42	2	4

170G	57g	203	45	2	4
180G	60g	213	47	2	5
190G	63g	224	50	2	5
200G	67g	238	53	2	5
210G	70g	249	55	2	6
220G	73g	260	57	3	6
230G	77g	274	61	3	6
240G	80g	284	63	3	6
250G	83g	295	65	3	7
260G	87g	309	68	3	7
270G	90g	320	71	3	7
280G	93g	331	73	3	7
290G	97g	345	76	3	7
300G	100g	355	78	3	8

Brown rice

C WEIGHT	UC WEIGHT	CALORIES	CARBS	FAT	PROTEIN
5G	1.7g	3	1	0	0
10G	3g	6	1	0	0
20G	7g	12	3	0	0
25G	8g	14	3	0	0
30G	10g	18	4	0	0
40G	13g	23	5	0	0
50G	17g	30	6	0	0
60G	20g	35	7	0	0
70G	23g	40	8	0	0
75G	25g	43	9	1	0
80G	27g	47	9	1	0
90G	30g	˙52	10	1	0
100G	33g	57	11	1	1
110G	37g	64	13	1	1
120G	40g	69	14	1	1
130G	43g	74	15	1	1
140G	47g	81	16	1	1
150G	50g	86	17	1	1
160G	53g	91	18	2	1
170G	57g	98	19	2	1

180G	60g	103	20	2	1
190G	63g	108	21	2	2
200G	67g	115	22	2	2
210G	70g	120	23	2	2
220G	73g	125	24	2	2
230G	77g	132	26	2	2
240G	80g	137	27	2	2
250G	83g	142	28	2	2
260G	87g	149	29	2	2
270G	90g	154	30	2	2
280G	93g	160	31	2	3
290G	97g	166	32	2	3
300G	100g	171	33	2	3

Pasta

Pasta takes up a lot of water too, but not as much as rice. **Pasta's weight x 2.5 more by the end of the cooking process.** There is lots of different information online about it too, so I measured, cooked as per instruction and calculated it. If your meal plan shows let's say 75g, then add up calories and macros by 70g+5g. If your meal plan does not show any pasta but you would like to eat some, you just need to match the calories and carbs. For example: if you can eat let's say 100g of cooked rice, that is 118Cal and 26C so instead of that you can eat 80g cooked pasta, that is 114Cal and 24C – which means your Cal is fine and you 'saved' 2C.

(C weight = Cooked weight; UC weight = Uncooked weight)

TIP: Read pasta labels very carefully when comparing types and brands. It does not always show the uncooked nutrition. Sometimes it says "Nutrition – when cooked according to instructions 100g" – 100g "cooked" means 40g uncooked!

C WEIGHT	UC WEIGHT	CALORIES	CARBS	FAT	PROTEIN
5G	2g	8	2	0	0
10G	4g	15	3	0	0
20G	8g	29	6	0	0
25G	10g	36	8	0	1
30G	12g	43	9	0	1
40G	16g	57	12	0	1
50G	20g	72	15	0	1
60G	24g	86	18	0	2
70G	28g	100	21	0	2
75G	30g	107	22	0	3
80G	32g	114	24	0	3
90G	36g	129	26	1	4
100G	40g	143	29	1	4
110G	44g	157	32	1	5
120G	48g	171	35	1	5
130G	52g	186	38	1	6
140G	56g	200	41	1	6
150G	60g	214	44	1	7
160G	64g	228	47	1	7
170G	68g	243	49	2	8
180G	72g	257	52	2	8
190G	76g	271	55	2	9
200G	80g	285	58	2	9
210G	84g	300	61	2	10
220G	88g	314	64	2	10
230G	92g	328	67	2	11
240G	96g	342	70	2	11
250G	100g	356	72	2	12

*TIP: For **low-carb high protein** pasta, tortilla and bread, visit CarbZone. Their pasta has 5 times more protein and 5 times less carbs than regular pasta. 100g contains **324 Cal, 14C, 3F, 60P**- https://carbzone.co.uk/*

Wholegrain Pasta

C WEIGHT	UC WEIGHT	CALORIES	CARBS	FAT	PROTEIN
5G	2g	7	2	0	0
10G	4g	14	3	0	0
20G	8g	27	6	0	0
25G	10g	34	7	0	1
30G	12g	41	8	0	1
40G	16g	54	11	0	1
50G	20g	68	14	0	2
60G	24g	81	16	0	2
70G	28g	95	19	0	2
75G	30g	101	20	0	2
80G	32g	108	22	1	3
90G	36g	121	24	1	3
100G	40g	135	27	1	4
110G	44g	148	29	1	4
120G	48g	162	32	1	5
130G	52g	175	35	1	5
140G	56g	189	37	1	6
150G	60g	202	40	1	6
160G	64g	216	43	1	6
170G	68g	229	45	2	7
180G	72g	242	48	2	7
190G	76g	256	51	2	8
200G	80g	269	53	2	8
210G	84g	283	56	2	9
220G	88g	296	58	2	9
230G	92g	310	61	2	9
240G	96g	323	64	2	9
250G	100g	336	66	2	10

Potato

Try to avoid frozen wedges/fries because they are usually coated in butter, which means they contain a lot more calories, carbs and fat than homemade, air-fried, no oil wedges/fries.

	CALORIES	CARB	FAT	PROTEIN
5G	5	2	0	0
10G	9	3	0	0
20G	18	6	0	0
25G	22	7	0	0
30G	27	8	0	0
40G	35	11	0	0
50G	44	14	0	1
60G	53	16	0	1
70G	61	19	0	1
75G	66	20	0	1
80G	70	22	0	1
90G	79	24	0	2
100G	87	27	0	2
125G	109	34	0	2
150G	131	40	0	3
175G	153	47	0	4
200G	174	53	0	4
225G	200	60	0	5
250G	218	67	0	5
275G	240	73	0	6
300G	261	80	0	6

Sweet potato

	CALORIES	CARB	FAT	PROTEIN
5G	5	2	0	0
10G	10	3	0	0
20G	19	5	0	0
25G	23	6	0	0

91

30G	28	7	0	0
40G	37	9	0	0
50G	46	11	0	1
60G	56	13	0	1
70G	65	15	0	1
75G	69	16	0	1
80G	74	17	0	1
90G	83	19	0	2
100G	92	21	0	2
125G	115	27	0	2
150G	138	32	0	3
175G	161	37	0	4
200G	184	42	0	4
225G	207	48	0	5
250G	230	53	0	5
275G	253	58	0	6
300G	276	63	0	6

TIP: If you want to save some carbs, use konjac noodles/pasta/rice. Not everybody likes it because of its texture and some brand's konjac noodles smells fishy when you open the pack. Just follow the instructions and rinse them with some cold water. They do not need any cooking, which means you can add it to your salad too. After rinsing them they do NOT taste fishy. (If they did, I would never eat them, trust me!) Worth a try?

My favourite **konjac noodles** are called 'Barenaked'. 100g contains **12Cal, 1C, 0F, 0P**.

My favourite **konjac pasta** (they have spaghetti and penne style) are called 'Slim Pasta', 100g contains **35Cal, 9C, 0F, 0P**.

And my favourite "rice-style" **konjac rice** is called 'Saitaku', 100g contains **8Cal, 0C, 0F, 0P**.

My favourite sides

It is time for you to check the nutrition of your favourite sides and make a note here. Make sure your calories and carbs are matching your meal plan and mark any deficits on the side. Do this and you will know if you have any extra carbs left for your treat ☺.

Description	Weight/ amount	Calories	Carbs	Fat	Protein

Description	Weight/ amount	Calories	Carbs	Fat	Protein

Dairy

Please note, that apart from fat-free cottage cheese, low-fat Greek style yoghurt, low-fat quark or protein quark, I do not use any other dairy and **I do not recommend using it on a daily basis.**

I did include some here because you might need it for cooking, but please use as little as possible, or leave it out of the recipe altogether. If you use any cheese then make sure you adjust your fat intake on that particular day.

TIP: Always use 0% fat or low-fat products where possible.

Fat-free cottage cheese

	CALORIES	CARBS	FAT	PROTEIN
5G	4	1	0	0
10G	7	1	0	1
20G	13	1	0	2
25G	16	2	0	2
30G	19	2	0	3
40G	25	2	0	4
50G	31	3	0	5
60G	38	3	0	6
70G	44	4	0	7
75G	47	4	0	7
80G	50	4	0	8
90G	56	5	0	9
100G	62	5	0	10
125G	78	6	0	12
150G	93	8	0	15
175G	109	9	0	17
200G	124	10	0	20
225G	140	11	0	22
250G	155	12	0	25

0% fat Greek style yoghurt (Fage)

	CALORIES	CARBS	FAT	PROTEIN
5G	3	0	1	1
10G	6	1	0	1
20G	11	1	0	2
25G	14	1	0	2
30G	17	1	0	3
40G	22	2	0	4
50G	27	2	0	5
60G	33	2	0	6
70G	38	3	0	7
75G	41	3	0	7
80G	44	3	0	8
90G	49	3	0	9
100G	54	3	0	10
125G	68	4	0	12
150G	81	5	0	15
175G	95	6	0	18
200G	108	6	0	20
225G	122	7	0	23
250G	135	8	0	25

Fat-free quark (Tesco)

	CALORIES	CARBS	FAT	PROTEIN
5G	4	0	0	0
10G	7	1	0	1
20G	13	1	0	2
25G	16	1	0	2
30G	19	2	0	3
40G	26	2	0	4
50G	32	2	0	5
60G	38	3	0	6
70G	45	3	0	8

	CALORIES	CARBS	FAT	PROTEIN
75G	48	3	0	8
80G	51	3	0	9
90G	57	4	0	10
100G	63	4	0	11
125G	79	5	0	14
150G	95	6	0	17
175G	111	7	0	20
200G	126	7	0	23
225G	142	8	0	25
250G	158	9	0	28

Low fat, high protein quark (Arla)

	CALORIES	CARBS	FAT	PROTEIN
5G	4	1	0	0
10G	7	1	0	1
20G	14	2	0	2
25G	18	2	0	2
30G	21	3	0	3
40G	28	3	0	4
50G	35	4	0	5
60G	42	5	0	6
70G	49	5	0	7
75G	53	6	0	7
80G	56	6	0	8
90G	63	7	0	9
100G	70	7	0	10
125G	88	9	0	12
150G	105	11	0	15
175G	123	12	0	17
200G	140	14	0	20
225G	158	16	0	22
250G	175	17	0	25

Coconut spread (Koko)

	CALORIES	CARBS	FAT	PROTEIN
5G	21	0	3	0
10G	41	0	5	0
20G	81	0	9	0
25G	102	0	12	0
30G	122	0	14	0
40G	162	0	18	0
50G	203	0	23	0
60G	243	0	27	0
70G	283	0	32	0
75G	304	0	34	0
80G	324	0	36	0
90G	365	0	41	0
100G	405	0	45	0
125G	507	0	57	0
150G	608	0	68	0
175G	709	0	79	0
200G	810	0	90	0
225G	912	0	102	0
250G	1013	0	113	0

Philadelphia Light

	CALORIES	CARBS	FAT	PROTEIN
5G	8	1	1	0
10G	15	1	2	0
20G	30	2	3	1
25G	38	2	3	1
30G	45	2	4	2
40G	60	3	5	2
50G	75	3	6	3
60G	90	4	7	4
70G	105	4	8	5
75G	113	4	9	5
80G	120	5	9	5

	CALORIES	CARBS	FAT	PROTEIN
90G	135	5	10	6
100G	150	6	11	7
125G	188	7	14	9
150G	225	8	17	10
175G	263	10	20	12
200G	300	11	22	14
225G	338	12	25	16
250G	375	13	28	18

Mozzarella

	CALORIES	CARBS	FAT	PROTEIN
5G	15	0	1	0
10G	30	0	3	1
20G	60	1	5	3
25G	74	1	6	4
30G	89	1	7	5
40G	119	2	9	6
50G	148	2	11	8
60G	178	2	13	10
70G	208	3	16	11
75G	222	3	17	12
80G	237	3	18	13
90G	267	3	20	15
100G	296	3	22	17
125G	370	4	27	21
150G	444	5	33	25
175G	518	6	38	29
200G	592	6	43	34
225G	666	7	49	38
250G	740	8	54	43

Cheddar, Edam, Gouda

	CALORIES	CARBS	FAT	PROTEIN
5G	21	0	2	1
10G	42	0	4	2
20G	84	1	7	4
25G	104	1	9	5
30G	125	1	11	7
40G	167	1	14	9
50G	208	2	18	12
60G	250	2	21	14
70G	292	2	24	16
75G	312	2	26	17
80G	333	2	28	19
90G	375	2	31	21
100G	416	3	35	23
125G	520	3	43	29
150G	624	4	52	35
175G	728	4	60	41
200G	832	5	69	47
225G	936	5	77	53
250G	1040	6	86	59

Parmigiano Reggiano
(Parmesan – Italian hard cheese)

	CALORIES	CARBS	FAT	PROTEIN
5G	21	0	2	1
10G	41	0	3	3
20G	81	0	6	6
25G	101	0	8	8
30G	121	0	9	9
40G	161	0	12	12
50G	201	0	15	16
60G	242	0	18	19
70G	282	0	21	22
75G	302	0	23	24

	CALORIES	CARBS	FAT	PROTEIN
80G	322	0	24	25
90G	362	0	27	29
100G	402	0	30	32
125G	503	0	38	41
150G	603	0	45	48
175G	704	0	52	56
200G	804	0	60	64
225G	905	0	67	72
250G	1005	0	75	81

Paneer
(Indian cheese)

	CALORIES	CARBS	FAT	PROTEIN
5G	18	0	2	1
10G	35	0	3	2
20G	70	1	6	4
25G	87	2	7	5
30G	105	2	9	5
40G	139	2	12	8
50G	174	3	14	10
60G	209	3	17	12
70G	243	3	20	14
75G	261	4	21	15
80G	278	4	23	16
90G	313	4	25	19
100G	347	5	28	20
125G	434	6	35	26
150G	521	7	42	31
175G	608	8	49	36
200G	694	9	56	41
225G	781	10	63	47
250G	868	11	70	52

Light Feta
(Greek cheese)

	CALORIES	CARBS	FAT	PROTEIN
5G	9	0	1	0
10G	17	0	1	2
20G	33	1	2	3
25G	41	1	3	4
30G	49	1	3	4
40G	66	2	4	6
50G	82	2	5	8
60G	98	2	6	9
70G	115	3	7	11
75G	123	3	7	12
80G	131	3	8	13
90G	147	3	9	14
100G	163	4	10	16
125G	204	4	12	20
150G	245	5	14	24
175G	286	6	17	29
200G	326	7	19	33
225G	367	8	21	37
250G	408	8	24	41

Halloumi
(Medium fat hard cheese)

	CALORIES	CARBS	FAT	PROTEIN
5G	18	0	2	1
10G	35	0	3	2
20G	69	0	6	4
25G	86	0	7	5
30G	104	1	8	6
40G	138	1	11	8
50G	172	1	14	11
60G	207	2	16	13
70G	241	2	19	15

75G	258	2	20	16
80G	276	2	22	17
90G	310	2	24	19
100G	344	2	27	22
125G	430	3	34	27
150G	516	3	40	33
175G	602	4	47	38
200G	688	4	54	44
225G	774	5	60	49
250G	860	5	67	55

Ricotta

	CALORIES	CARBS	FAT	PROTEIN
5G	6	0	0	0
10G	11	0	1	0
20G	21	1	2	1
25G	26	1	2	1
30G	31	1	3	2
40G	42	2	3	2
50G	52	2	4	3
60G	62	2	5	4
70G	73	3	5	4
75G	78	3	6	5
80G	83	3	6	5
90G	93	3	7	6
100G	103	3	7	7
125G	129	4	9	8
150G	155	5	11	10
175G	181	6	13	12
200G	206	6	14	14
225G	232	7	16	15
250G	258	8	18	17

Mascarpone

	CALORIES	CARBS	FAT	PROTEIN
5G	22	0	3	0
10G	44	0	5	0
20G	87	1	9	1
25G	109	1	11	1
30G	131	2	14	1
40G	174	2	18	2
50G	217	2	22	3
60G	261	3	27	3
70G	304	3	31	4
75G	326	3	33	4
80G	348	3	36	4
90G	391	4	40	5
100G	434	4	44	6
125G	543	5	55	7
150G	651	6	66	9
175G	760	7	77	10
200G	868	7	88	12
225G	977	8	99	14
250G	1085	9	110	15

Soured cream

	CALORIES	CARBS	FAT	PROTEIN
5G	10	1	1	0
10G	20	1	2	0
20G	39	1	4	0
25G	48	2	5	0
30G	58	2	6	0
40G	75	2	8	0
50G	96	3	10	1
60G	115	3	12	1
70G	134	3	13	1
75G	144	4	14	1
80G	153	4	15	1

	CALORIES	CARBS	FAT	PROTEIN
90G	172	4	17	2
100G	191	5	19	2
125G	239	6	24	2
150G	287	7	28	3
175G	335	8	33	4
200G	382	9	37	4
225G	430	10	42	5
250G	478	11	47	5

Crème Fraiche

(Use soured cream instead of crème fraiche)

	CALORIES	CARBS	FAT	PROTEIN
5G	16	0	2	0
10G	31	0	4	0
20G	61	1	7	0
25G	76	1	8	0
30G	91	1	10	0
40G	121	2	13	0
50G	151	2	16	1
60G	182	2	19	1
70G	212	2	22	1
75G	227	3	24	2
80G	242	3	25	2
90G	272	3	28	2
100G	302	3	32	2
125G	378	4	39	3
150G	453	5	47	4
175G	529	5	55	4
200G	604	6	63	5
225G	680	7	70	6
250G	750	7	78	6

Single cream

	CALORIES	CARBS	FAT	PROTEIN
5G	8	0	1	0
10G	16	1	2	0
20G	32	1	3	0
25G	40	2	4	0
30G	48	2	5	0
40G	64	2	6	1
50G	80	3	8	1
60G	96	3	9	1
70G	112	4	11	2
75G	120	4	12	2
80G	128	4	12	2
90G	144	5	14	2
100G	159	5	15	3
125G	199	6	19	3
150G	239	7	23	4
175G	279	8	27	5
200G	318	9	30	6
225G	358	11	33	6
250G	398	12	38	7

Double cream

(Use single cream instead of double cream)

	CALORIES	CARBS	FAT	PROTEIN
5G	17	0	2	0
10G	34	1	4	0
20G	67	1	7	0
25G	84	1	9	0
30G	101	2	11	0
40G	134	2	14	0
50G	168	2	18	1
60G	201	3	21	1
70G	235	3	25	1
75G	252	3	27	1

	CALORIES	CARBS	FAT	PROTEIN
80G	268	4	28	1
90G	302	4	32	1
100G	335	4	35	2
125G	419	5	44	2
150G	503	6	53	3
175G	587	7	62	4
200G	670	8	70	4
225G	754	9	79	5
250G	838	10	88	5

Half-fat curd cheese

	CALORIES	CARBS	FAT	PROTEIN
5G	6	0	0	0
10G	12	1	1	1
20G	23	1	1	3
25G	28	1	1	4
30G	34	2	2	4
40G	45	2	2	6
50G	56	2	2	8
60G	67	3	3	9
70G	78	3	3	11
75G	84	3	3	12
80G	89	4	3	12
90G	100	4	4	14
100G	112	4	4	16
125G	139	5	5	20
150G	167	6	6	24
175G	195	7	7	28
200G	222	8	7	32
225G	250	9	8	36
250G	278	10	9	40

Reduced-fat coconut cream

	CALORIES	CARBS	FAT	PROTEIN
5G	5	0	1	0
10G	9	0	1	0
20G	18	0	2	0
25G	22	1	3	0
30G	26	1	3	0
40G	35	1	4	0
50G	43	1	5	0
60G	52	1	6	0
70G	61	1	7	0
75G	65	1	7	0
80G	69	1	8	0
90G	75	1	9	0
100G	86	2	9	0
125G	108	2	12	0
150G	129	2	14	0
175G	151	2	16	0
200G	172	3	18	0
225G	194	3	20	0
250G	215	3	23	0

Coconut cream
(Use reduced fat coconut cream)

	CALORIES	CARBS	FAT	PROTEIN
5G	11	0	2	0
10G	22	0	3	0
20G	44	1	5	0
25G	55	1	6	0
30G	66	1	7	0
40G	88	2	9	0
50G	109	2	11	0
60G	131	2	14	0
70G	153	2	16	0
75G	164	2	17	0

80G	175	3	18	0
90G	197	3	20	0
100G	218	3	22	1
125G	273	4	28	1
150G	327	4	33	1
175G	382	5	39	1
200G	436	6	44	2
225G	491	6	50	2
250G	545	7	55	2

My favourite dairy/cheese

Description	Weight/ amount	Calories	Carbs	Fat	Protein

Sauces, dips and dressings

For cooking

Chopped tomatoes in tomato juice

	CALORIES	CARBS	FAT	PROTEIN
5G	1	0	0	0
10G	2	0	0	0
25G	5	1	0	0
50G	9	2	0	0
75G	14	3	0	0
100G	18	3	0	1
125G	23	4	0	1
150G	27	5	0	1
175G	32	6	0	1
200G	36	6	0	2
225G	41	7	0	2
250G	45	8	0	2
275G	50	9	0	2
300G	54	9	0	3
325G	59	10	0	3
350G	63	11	0	3
375G	68	12	0	3
400G	72	12	0	4
425G	77	13	0	4
450G	81	14	0	4
475G	86	15	0	4
500G	90	15	0	5

Dolmio Bolognese sauce

	CALORIES	CARBS	FAT	PROTEIN
5G	3	1	0	0
10G	5	1	0	0
25G	13	3	0	0
50G	25	5	0	0
75G	38	7	1	1
100G	50	9	1	1
125G	63	11	1	2
150G	75	13	2	2
175G	85	12	2	2
200G	100	17	2	3
225G	113	19	2	3
250G	125	21	2	4
275G	138	23	2	4
300G	150	25	3	4
325G	163	27	3	5
350G	175	29	3	5
375G	188	31	3	6
400G	200	33	3	6
425G	213	35	3	7
450G	225	37	4	7
475G	238	39	4	7
500G	250	41	4	8

Black bean sauce

	CALORIES	CARBS	FAT	PROTEIN
5G	8	1	0	0
10G	15	2	0	0
20G	29	4	0	1
30G	44	6	1	2
40G	58	7	2	3
50G	72	9	2	4
60G	87	12	3	5
70G	101	12	3	6

Hoisin sauce

	CALORIES	CARBS	FAT	PROTEIN
5G	12	3	0	0
10G	23	6	0	0
20G	46	11	0	0
30G	69	16	0	0
40G	92	22	0	0
50G	114	27	0	0
60G	137	32	1	1
70G	160	38	1	1

Teriyaki sauce

	CALORIES	CARBS	FAT	PROTEIN
5G	12	3	0	0
10G	23	5	0	0
20G	46	9	1	0
30G	69	14	1	1
40G	92	18	2	1
50G	114	22	2	2
60G	137	27	2	2
70G	160	31	2	3

Soy sauce

	CALORIES	CARBS	FAT	PROTEIN
5G	4	0	0	0
10G	8	1	0	1
15G	12	1	0	1
20G	16	1	0	2
25G	20	1	0	2
30G	24	1	0	3
35G	27	2	0	3
40G	31	2	0	4
45G	35	2	0	4
50G	39	2	0	5

I very rarely use sauces, dips or dressings. **I do not recommend using any!** You can save lots of calories, carbs and fat by avoiding it. I included some below – only the fat-free versions where available! **Always look for the reduced fat/sugar varieties.**

Serving size: 15g (1 tbsp)

Sweet Chilli sauce

	CALORIES	CARBS	FAT	PROTEIN
15G – 1 SERVING	24	6	0	0
30G – 2 SERVING	47	12	0	0
45G – 3 SERVING	70	17	0	0
60G- 4 SERVING	92	23	0	0
75G – 5 SERVING	116	28	0	0

Raita

	CALORIES	CARBS	FAT	PROTEIN
15G – 1 SERVING	31	1	3	0
30G – 2 SERVING	71	2	6	0
45G –	92	3	9	0

3 SERVING				
60G- 4 SERVING	122	3	12	0
75G – 5 SERVING	153	4	15	1

Mango chutney

	CALORIES	CARBS	FAT	PROTEIN
15G – 1 SERVING	36	9	0	0
30G – 2 SERVING	71	17	0	0
45G – 3 SERVING	106	26	0	0
60G- 4 SERVING	141	34	0	0
75G – 5 SERVING	176	43	0	0

Reduced fat houmous

	CALORIES	CARBS	FAT	PROTEIN
15G – 1 SERVING	26	2	2	0
30G – 2 SERVING	51	4	3	1

45G – 3 SERVING	76	6	5	2
60G- 4 SERVING	101	8	6	3
75G – 5 SERVING	126	10	7	4

Guacamole

	CALORIES	CARBS	FAT	PROTEIN
15G – 1 SERVING	20	0	2	0
30G – 2 SERVING	39	1	4	0
45G – 3 SERVING	59	1	6	0
60G- 4 SERVING	79	2	8	0
75G – 5 SERVING	98	2	10	1

Tzatziki

	CALORIES	CARBS	FAT	PROTEIN
15G – 1 SERVING	18	1	2	0
30G – 2 SERVING	36	2	3	1

	CALORIES	CARBS	FAT	PROTEIN
45G – 3 SERVING	54	3	5	1
60G- 4 SERVING	72	3	6	2
75G – 5 SERVING	90	4	8	2

Onion and garlic dip

	CALORIES	CARBS	FAT	PROTEIN
15G – 1 SERVING	37	1	4	0
30G – 2 SERVING	73	2	8	0
45G – 3 SERVING	110	3	11	0
60G- 4 SERVING	146	4	15	1
75G – 5 SERVING	183	5	18	1

Soured cream and chive dip

	CALORIES	CARBS	FAT	PROTEIN
15G – 1 SERVING	35	1	4	0
30G – 2 SERVING	70	2	7	0

	CALORIES	CARBS	FAT	PROTEIN
45G – 3 SERVING	104	3	10	0
60G- 4 SERVING	139	4	14	1
75G – 5 SERVING	174	5	17	1

Low-fat Heinz salad cream

	CALORIES	CARBS	FAT	PROTEIN
15G – 1 SERVING	34	3	3	0
30G – 2 SERVING	67	5	5	0
45G – 3 SERVING	100	7	8	0
60G- 4 SERVING	133	9	10	0
75G – 5 SERVING	166	11	13	0

Classic BBQ Heinz

	CALORIES	CARBS	FAT	PROTEIN
15G – 1 SERVING	21	6	0	0
30G – 2 SERVING	42	11	0	0

	CALORIES	CARBS	FAT	PROTEIN
45G – 3 SERVING	63	16	0	0
60G- 4 SERVING	83	21	0	0
75G – 5 SERVING	104	26	0	0

Tartare sauce

	CALORIES	CARBS	FAT	PROTEIN
15G – 1 SERVING	56	3	5	0
30G – 2 SERVING	111	6	10	0
45G – 3 SERVING	167	9	15	0
60G- 4 SERVING	222	12	20	0
75G – 5 SERVING	277	15	25	0

Mint sauce

	CALORIES	CARBS	FAT	PROTEIN
15G – 1 SERVING	18	4	0	0
30G – 2 SERVING	36	8	0	0

	CALORIES	CARBS	FAT	PROTEIN
45G – 3 SERVING	54	12	0	0
60G- 4 SERVING	72	15	0	1
75G – 5 SERVING	90	19	0	1

Bramley apple sauce

	CALORIES	CARBS	FAT	PROTEIN
15G – 1 SERVING	16	4	0	0
30G – 2 SERVING	32	8	0	0
45G – 3 SERVING	48	12	0	0
60G- 4 SERVING	64	15	0	0
75G – 5 SERVING	80	20	0	0

50% less sugar and salt Ketchup Heinz

	CALORIES	CARBS	FAT	PROTEIN
15G – 1 SERVING	10	2	0	0
30G – 2 SERVING	20	4	0	0

	CALORIES	CARBS	FAT	PROTEIN
45G – 3 SERVING	29	6	0	0
60G- 4 SERVING	39	8	0	0
75G – 5 SERVING	48	9	0	1

Lighter than light mayonnaise Hellmann's

	CALORIES	CARBS	FAT	PROTEIN
15G – 1 SERVING	11	2	1	0
30G – 2 SERVING	22	3	1	0
45G – 3 SERVING	33	5	2	0
60G- 4 SERVING	44	6	2	0
75G – 5 SERVING	54	7	3	0

Reduced sugar and salt brown sauce

	CALORIES	CARBS	FAT	PROTEIN
15G – 1 SERVING	11	3	0	0
30G – 2 SERVING	21	5	0	0

	CALORIES	CARBS	FAT	PROTEIN
45G – 3 SERVING	32	8	0	0
60G- 4 SERVING	42	10	0	0
75G – 5 SERVING	53	12	0	0

Garlic and herb sauce Hellmann's

	CALORIES	CARBS	FAT	PROTEIN
15G – 1 SERVING	43	2	4	0
30G – 2 SERVING	85	4	8	0
45G – 3 SERVING	128	6	12	0
60G- 4 SERVING	170	8	15	0
75G – 5 SERVING	213	10	19	0

American style burger sauce Heinz

	CALORIES	CARBS	FAT	PROTEIN
15G – 1 SERVING	57	2	6	0
30G – 2 SERVING	113	4	11	0

	CALORIES	CARBS	FAT	PROTEIN
45G – 3 SERVING	169	6	17	0
60G- 4 SERVING	226	8	22	0
75G – 5 SERVING	282	9	27	0

Mayo-Ketchup sauce Heinz

	CALORIES	CARBS	FAT	PROTEIN
15G – 1 SERVING	65	3	7	0
30G – 2 SERVING	130	5	13	0
45G – 3 SERVING	195	7	19	0
60G- 4 SERVING	260	9	25	0
75G – 5 SERVING	324	11	31	0

Mustard

	CALORIES	CARBS	FAT	PROTEIN
15G – 1 SERVING	16	2	1	0
30G – 2 SERVING	32	3	2	1

	CALORIES	CARBS	FAT	PROTEIN
45G – 3 SERVING	48	5	3	2
60G- 4 SERVING	63	6	4	2
75G – 5 SERVING	79	7	4	3

Chilli sauce

	CALORIES	CARBS	FAT	PROTEIN
15G – 1 SERVING	22	5	0	0
30G – 2 SERVING	43	9	0	0
45G – 3 SERVING	64	14	0	0
60G- 4 SERVING	85	18	1	1
75G – 5 SERVING	106	23	1	1

Thousand Island dressing

	CALORIES	CARBS	FAT	PROTEIN
15G – 1 SERVING	45	3	4	0
30G – 2 SERVING	89	5	8	0

	CALORIES	CARBS	FAT	PROTEIN
45G – 3 SERVING	133	7	12	0
60G- 4 SERVING	177	10	16	0
75G – 5 SERVING	222	12	19	0

Caesar dressing

	CALORIES	CARBS	FAT	PROTEIN
15G – 1 SERVING	59	1	7	0
30G – 2 SERVING	118	2	13	0
45G – 3 SERVING	177	3	19	0
60G- 4 SERVING	236	3	25	0
75G – 5 SERVING	295	4	31	0

Reduced fat French dressing

	CALORIES	CARBS	FAT	PROTEIN
15G – 1 SERVING	10	2	0	0
30G – 2 SERVING	20	4	0	0

125

45G – 3 SERVING	30	6	1	0
60G- 4 SERVING	39	8	1	0
75G – 5 SERVING	49	10	1	0

TIP: Try some guilt-free zero sauces from Skinny Food Co. – https://theskinnyfoodco.com/ They have lots of choice. Do not expect the exact same taste as the original sauce though…

My favourite sauce/dip/dressing

Description	Weight/ amount	Calories	Carbs	Fat	Protein

My lunch + dinner calories and macros

Before creating your lunch/dinner meals, the best thing to do is to calculate and write down your lunch + dinner calories and macros so you do not have to calculate it over and over again. This is only your lunch + dinner macros, not the whole day.

	Calories	Carbs	Fat	Protein
For 1 day				
For 2 days				
For 3 days				
For 4 days				
For 5 days				
For 6 days				
For 7 days				

Learn how to create your recipe that matches your calories and macros

Ta-da! It is time for you to create your own recipe and I'll show you how, step-by-step.

I am also sharing one of my favourite recipes here ☺. It is very quick and yummy, it is called 'Fasirt' – it is a type of Hungarian meatball.

Example: (please note, these are NOT my macros, it's totally made up for this example)

1. Check your daily lunch/dinner macros. Let's say it is: 470Cal, 45C, 15F, 45P

2. Let's start with the **fixed amounts**.

   Let's say you have 70g cooked rice on your meal plan and 130g beef, so that's given. You will add them up and calculate those two first, they are in your tables above. This is for 1 day.

   70g rice: 81Cal, 20C, 0F, 1P
   130g minced beef: 162Cal, 0C, 7F, 28P
   Total: 243Cal, 20C, 7F, 29P

3. Based on this, calculate what you have **left**.

   You have 227Cal, 25C, 8F left and you need 16g more protein.

4. Decide how many days you are cooking for.

   Let's say you are cooking for the next 3 days.
   So you can use 3 times of what you have left, it will be:

681Cal, 75C, 24F and you need to make up 48g of protein.

5. Now have a look at the **original recipe**.

   1000g minced pork or 500g minced pork and 500g minced beef
   200g onion
   6 garlic cloves, crushed
   150g breadcrumb
   125g parsley
   3 whole eggs
   1 tsp paprika powder
   salt
   pepper

6. **Amend it** to fit your macros.

   Your meat is given and calculated already, so you know it's 390g for 3 days (you need to cook 489g).

   You will adjust the onion, because it is for 1000g of meat and we are using 489g, which is less than half. We will use 100g. You know from your table, that it is 40Cal, 9C, 0F, 1P. You have **641Cal** and **66C** left and need to **make up for 47g protein**.

   We adjust the garlic too, we are using half of the meat, so we will use half of the garlic, which means 3 cloves of garlic. It is 12Cal, 3C, 0F, 0P. You have **629Cal** and **63C** left.

   We will of course adjust the breadcrumbs too, way too many carbs... This meatball is supposed to be breadcrumbed and deep fried. Now it will not be breadcrumbed and will not be deep fried. You will bake it in the oven on baking paper or in an air-fryer using zero oil. We still need to use a little bit of breadcrumbs, they soak up some of the juice that comes out of the meat, so we will use 50g of breadcrumbs – 183Cal, 38C, 1F, 1P. (Check the nutrition info at the back of the pack!) You now have **446Cal, 25C** and **23F** left and need to **make up for 43g protein**.

We will add some parsley, about 4tbsp (16g) parsley, that is 6Cal, 1C. (**440Cal** and **24C** left)

The recipe says to use 3 whole eggs but we want to save carbs and make up for protein. So the aim is: lowest carb with highest protein. If you check your table, you will see it's 1 whole egg and 4 egg whites and it is 250Cal, 1C, 5F, 30P. You only need to add some spices after this. A little paprika powder and some salt and pepper to season – which is an insignificant amount in terms of calories and macros.

Your amended recipe will look like this:
Total for 3 days: 977Cal, 52C, 27F, 116P
Per day: 325Cal, 18C, 9F, 39P
488g minced beef
100g onion
3 garlic cloves, crushed
50g breadcrumbs (It tastes better with a little breadcrumb but it is not essential)
4tbsp finely chopped parsley
1 whole egg + 4 egg whites
1 tsp paprika powder
pepper
salt

Mix the ingredients well together in a bowl. Create balls and oven-bake or air-fry. You can also put your mix in a baking tray with some baking paper under it and oven-bake it. Have rice as a side. When your rice is ready, add and stir in 1 tbsp of parsley, it gives a great taste to your rice ☺.

How to adjust other macros

Let's say you want to cook for 3 days, you adjust your chosen recipe and you finish on: 20 Cal over, 35C over, 18F under and 36P under. That is for 3 days, which is: 7Cal over, 12C over, 6F under and 12P under per day.

You need to adjust this. 7Cal up or down is nothing really, you can live with that.

12g carb extra is no good, you can easily amend that by eating less fruit on those 3 given days. Fruit contains a lot of carbs. Also, you can use 10g less oats for your porridge or no toast on those 3 days.

6g fat is still missing, that is no good either, you can easily adjust this by eating about 5g more nuts on those 3 days.

And we were also missing 12g protein. I mean, add a little bit more protein powder to your shake ☺ (yes, that will add to your calories too but remember, we are lowering the amount of fruits already, so it will be fine).

After adjusting your other meals of the day, write down what and how much to have for your other meal, eg. for breakfast, more protein powder in your shake, more nuts, no snack, rice as side, etc.

Make sure you write it all down, because now you have a set meal plan that will cover 3 days (or even six days if you double it up) and you do not have to calculate anything again.

Please remember…

If you are about 10-50Cal +/- a day, it's okay.
If you are 1-7g carb +/- a day, it's okay.
If you are 1-3g fat +/- a day, it's okay.
If you are 1-3g protein +/- a day, it's okay (with protein, it is better to be a bit up than a bit down).

Of course, try to be **as close as possible**!
But do not beat yourself up over it if you are a tiny bit under or over.

Learn about your sources so you can easily adjust

To be able to make adjustments on your meal plan and get creative with it, you need to know the best sources to adjust.

PROTEIN SOURCES	CARB SOURCES	FAT SOURCES
Chicken breast	Rice	Avocado
Protein powder	Pasta	Oil
Fish (tuna and cod)	Potato	Nuts
Egg whites	Sweet potato	Egg yolk
	Bread	Cheese
	Oat	Olives
	Cereal	
	Fruits	
	Vegetables	
	Sauces,dips, dressings	

TIP: If you need to take carbs away, do it in this order: sauces/dips/dressings, bread, cereal, pasta/potato.

Now it is time to put your knowledge into practice and adjust 5-10 of your favourite recipe's to fit your calories and macros. I'll leave space for 10 recipes on the next few pages. Do it one-by-one. If you choose to then you can but you do not have to do 10 recipes right now. Do one a day and it will not be so overwhelming. Make sure you note anything you need to be careful with if you use that recipe, eg. "High fat, do not eat nuts", "Low protein, add more protein powder"

Now just create one or two so you have something to start with – be creative!

After that we will move onto fruits and treats.

My favourite recipes

Name:_____

Ingredients	Weight/ amount	Calories	Carbs	Fat	Protein

Total:					

Method:

Note for myself:

Name:_____

Ingredients	Weight/ amount	Calories	Carbs	Fat	Protein

Total:					

Method:

Note for myself:

Name:_____

Ingredients	Weight/amount	Calories	Carbs	Fat	Protein

Total:				

Method:

Note for myself:

Name:_____

Ingredients	Weight/ amount	Calories	Carbs	Fat	Protein

Total:					

Method:

Note for myself:

Name:_____

Ingredients	Weight/ amount	Calories	Carbs	Fat	Protein

Total:					

Method:

Note for myself:

Name:_____

Ingredients	Weight/ amount	Calories	Carbs	Fat	Protein

Total:					

Method:

Note for myself:

Name:_____

Ingredients	Weight/ amount	Calories	Carbs	Fat	Protein

Total:				

Method:

Note for myself:

Name:_____

Ingredients	Weight/amount	Calories	Carbs	Fat	Protein

Total:				

Method:

Note for myself:

Name:_____

Ingredients	Weight/ amount	Calories	Carbs	Fat	Protein

Total:				

Method:

Note for myself:

Name:_____

Ingredients	Weight/ amount	Calories	Carbs	Fat	Protein

Total:					

Method:

Note for myself:

Others

Avocado

	CALORIES	CARBS	FAT	PROTEIN
5G	8	1	1	0
10G	16	1	2	0
20G	32	2	4	0
25G	40	3	5	0
30G	48	3	6	0
40G	64	4	7	0
50G	80	5	9	1
60G	96	6	11	1
70G	112	7	12	1
75G	120	8	13	1
80G	128	8	14	1
90G	144	9	16	1
100G	160	10	17	2
125G	200	13	22	2
150G	240	15	26	3
175G	280	18	30	3
200G	320	20	34	4
300G	480	30	51	8

Peanut butter

	CALORIES	CARBS	FAT	PROTEIN
5G	29	1	3	1
10G	58	2	5	3
15G	87	2	7	4
20G	116	3	10	6
25G	145	3	12	7
30G	174	4	14	9
35G	203	5	17	10
40G	232	5	19	12
45G	261	6	21	13
50G	290	6	23	15
55G	319	7	26	16

60G	348	8	28	18
65G	377	8	30	19
70G	406	9	33	21
75G	435	9	35	22
80G	464	10	37	24
85G	493	11	40	25
90G	522	11	42	27
95G	551	12	44	29
100G	579	12	46	30

Coconut

	CALORIES	CARBS	FAT	PROTEIN
5G	15	1	2	0
10G	29	1	3	0
20G	57	2	6	0
25G	71	3	7	0
30G	85	3	9	0
35G	100	4	10	1
40G	114	4	11	1
45G	128	5	13	1
50G	142	5	14	1
55G	156	6	15	1
60G	170	6	17	1
65G	184	7	18	1
70G	199	7	19	2
75G	213	8	21	2
80G	227	8	22	2
85G	241	9	23	2
90G	255	9	25	2
95G	269	10	26	2
100G	283	10	27	3
125G	354	13	34	3
150G	425	14	41	4
175G	496	18	48	4
200G	566	20	54	6

Nuts

The nutrition in nuts is very similar, therefore I used the average calories, carbs, fat and protein content of 7 different nuts for the table below.

	CALORIES	CARBS	FAT	PROTEIN
5G	33	1	3	0
10G	66	1	6	1
15G	99	2	9	2
20G	132	2	12	3
25G	165	2	15	4
30G	198	3	18	5
35G	231	3	21	6
40G	264	4	24	6
45G	297	4	24	7
50G	330	4	30	8
55G	363	5	33	9
60G	396	5	36	10
65G	429	6	39	11
70G	462	6	42	12
75G	495	6	45	12
80G	528	7	48	13
85G	561	7	51	14
90G	594	8	54	15
95G	627	8	57	16
100G	660	8	60	17

Olives

	CALORIES	CARBS	FAT	PROTEIN
1 OLIVE	7	0	1	0
2 OLIVES	14	0	2	0
3 OLIVES	21	0	3	0
4 OLIVES	28	0	4	0
5 OLIVES	35	0	5	0
6 OLIVES	42	0	6	0
7 OLIVES	49	0	7	0
8 OLIVES	56	0	8	0
9 OLIVES	63	0	9	0
10 OLIVES	70	0	10	0

Chia seeds

	CALORIES	CARBS	FAT	PROTEIN
1 SERVING	67	1	6	3
2 SERVING	134	2	12	6
3 SERVING	201	3	18	9
4 SERVING	268	4	24	12
5 SERVING	335	5	30	15

*Serving size 15g

Kallo Rice cake

	CALORIES	CARBS	FAT	PROTEIN
1 SLICE	27	6	0	0
2 SLICES	54	12	1	1
3 SLICES	81	17	1	1
4 SLICES	108	23	1	2
5 SLICES	135	28	1	3

Tortilla wrap

	CALORIES	CARBS	FAT	PROTEIN
1 WRAP	173	31	4	5
2 WRAPS	346	61	7	10
3 WRAPS	519	91	10	15
4 WRAPS	692	122	13	20
5 WRAPS	865	152	16	25

*TIP: For **low-carb high protein** pasta, tortilla and bread, visit CarbZone. Their large tortilla wrap contains 200Cal, 7C, 9F, 14P/wrap. - https://carbzone.co.uk/*

Vegetable/Beef/Chicken stock

	CALORIES	CARBS	FAT	PROTEIN
1 SERVING	30	4	2	0
2 SERVING	60	8	4	0
3 SERVING	90	12	6	0
4 SERVING	120	16	8	0
5 SERVING	150	20	10	0

*Serving size = 1 cube

Coconut flour

	CALORIES	CARBS	FAT	PROTEIN
1 TBSP	36	2	2	0
2 TBSP	72	4	4	0
3 TBSP	108	6	6	0
4 TBSP	144	8	8	0
5 TBSP	180	10	10	0

*A tablespoon of flour is about 10g

159

Plain flour

	CALORIES	CARBS	FAT	PROTEIN
1 TBSP	37	8	0	0
2 TBSP	74	16	1	0
3 TBSP	111	24	2	0
4 TBSP	148	32	3	0
5 TBSP	185	40	4	0

*A tablespoon of flour is about 10g

Fruits

You will probably have some fruit on your meal plan. Make sure you match your calories and carbs as close as possible.

Lemon juice (raw)

	CALORIES	CARBS	FAT	PROTEIN
½ TBSP	2	0	0	0
1 TBSP	4	1	0	0
2 TBSP	8	2	0	0
3 TBSP	12	3	0	0

*An average lemon has about 2tbsp of juice

Lemon zest

	CALORIES	CARBS	FAT	PROTEIN
½ TBSP	2	0	0	0
1 TBSP	3	1	0	0
2 TBSP	6	2	0	0
3 TBSP	9	3	0	0

*An average lemon has about 1tbsp of zest

Lime juice (raw)

	CALORIES	CARBS	FAT	PROTEIN
½ TBSP	2	1	0	0
1 TBSP	4	2	0	0
2 TBSP	8	3	0	0
3 TBSP	12	4	0	0

*An average lime has about 2tbsp of juice

Strawberry

	CALORIES	CARBS	FAT	PROTEIN
5G	2	1	0	0
10G	4	1	0	0
20G	7	2	0	0
25G	8	2	0	0
30G	10	3	0	0
40G	13	4	0	0
50G	16	4	0	0
60G	20	5	0	0
70G	23	6	0	0
75G	24	6	0	0
80G	26	7	0	0
90G	29	7	0	0
100G	32	8	0	0
125G	40	10	0	0
150G	48	12	0	1
175G	56	14	1	1
200G	64	16	1	1
300G	96	24	1	2
400G	128	31	1	2
500G	160	39	1	3
600G	192	47	2	4

Raspberry

	CALORIES	CARBS	FAT	PROTEIN
5G	3	1	0	0
10G	6	2	0	0
20G	11	3	0	0
25G	13	3	0	0
30G	16	4	0	0
40G	21	5	0	0
50G	26	6	0	0
60G	32	8	0	0
70G	37	9	0	0

	CALORIES	CARBS	FAT	PROTEIN
75G	40	9	1	0
80G	42	10	1	0
90G	47	11	1	1
100G	52	12	1	1
125G	65	15	1	1
150G	78	18	2	1
175G	91	21	2	2
200G	104	24	2	2
300G	156	36	3	3
400G	208	48	3	4
500G	260	60	4	6
600G	312	72	5	7

Blueberry

	CALORIES	CARBS	FAT	PROTEIN
5G	3	1	0	0
10G	6	2	0	0
20G	12	3	0	0
25G	15	4	0	0
30G	18	5	0	0
40G	23	6	0	0
50G	29	7	0	0
60G	35	9	0	0
70G	40	10	0	0
75G	43	11	0	0
80G	46	12	0	0
90G	52	13	0	0
100G	57	14	0	0
125G	72	18	0	0
150G	86	21	0	1
175G	100	25	0	1
200G	118	28	1	1
300G	171	42	1	2
400G	228	56	2	2
500G	285	70	2	3
600G	342	84	2	4

Banana

	CALORIES	CARBS	FAT	PROTEIN
¼ BANANA	30	8	0	0
½ BANANA	59	16	0	0
¾ BANANA	89	23	0	1
1 BANANA	116	30	1	1
2 BANANAS	232	60	1	2
3 BANANAS	348	90	2	4
4 BANANAS	463	120	2	5
5 BANANAS	579	150	2	7

*Average weight of a banana is about 130g

Apple

	CALORIES	CARBS	FAT	PROTEIN
5G	3	1	0	0
10G	6	2	0	0
20G	12	3	0	0
25G	15	4	0	0
30G	18	5	0	0
40G	24	6	0	0
50G	29	7	0	0
60G	35	9	0	0
70G	41	10	0	0
75G	44	11	0	0
80G	47	12	0	0
90G	53	13	0	0
100G	58	14	0	0
125G	73	18	0	0
150G	87	21	0	0
175G	102	25	0	0

	CALORIES	CARBS	FAT	PROTEIN
200G	116	28	0	0
300G	174	42	0	1
400G	232	56	1	1
500G	290	70	1	2
600G	348	84	2	2

Pear

	CALORIES	CARBS	FAT	PROTEIN
5G	3	1	0	0
10G	6	2	0	0
20G	12	4	0	0
25G	15	4	0	0
30G	18	5	0	0
40G	24	7	0	0
50G	29	8	0	0
60G	35	10	0	0
70G	41	11	0	0
75G	44	12	0	0
80G	47	13	0	0
90G	53	14	0	0
100G	58	16	0	0
125G	73	20	0	0
150G	87	24	0	0
175G	102	28	0	0
200G	116	31	0	0
300G	174	47	0	1
400G	232	62	0	1
500G	290	78	0	2
600G	348	93	0	2

Peach

	CALORIES	CARBS	FAT	PROTEIN
5G	2	1	0	0
10G	4	1	0	0

	CALORIES	CARBS	FAT	PROTEIN
20G	8	2	0	0
25G	10	3	0	0
30G	12	3	0	0
40G	16	4	0	0
50G	20	5	0	0
60G	24	6	0	0
70G	28	7	0	0
75G	30	8	0	0
80G	32	8	0	0
90G	36	9	0	0
100G	39	10	0	0
125G	49	12	0	1
150G	59	15	0	1
175G	69	17	0	1
200G	78	20	1	1
300G	118	29	1	2
400G	156	39	1	3
500G	195	48	2	4
600G	234	58	2	5

Orange

	CALORIES	CARBS	FAT	PROTEIN
5G	3	1	0	0
10G	5	2	0	0
20G	10	3	0	0
25G	13	4	0	0
30G	15	4	0	0
40G	20	6	0	0
50G	25	7	0	0
60G	30	8	0	0
70G	35	10	0	0
75G	37	10	0	0
80G	40	11	0	0
90G	45	12	0	0
100G	49	13	0	0
125G	62	17	0	0
150G	74	20	0	1

	CALORIES	CARBS	FAT	PROTEIN
175G	86	23	0	1
200G	98	26	0	1
300G	147	39	0	2
400G	196	52	0	3
500G	245	65	1	4
600G	294	78	1	5

Clementine

	CALORIES	CARBS	FAT	PROTEIN
5G	3	1	0	0
10G	5	2	0	0
20G	10	3	0	0
25G	12	3	0	0
30G	15	4	0	0
40G	19	5	0	0
50G	24	6	0	0
60G	29	8	0	0
70G	33	9	0	0
75G	36	9	0	0
80G	38	10	0	0
90G	43	11	0	0
100G	47	12	0	0
125G	59	15	0	0
150G	71	18	0	1
175G	83	21	0	1
200G	94	24	0	1
300G	141	36	0	2
400G	188	48	0	3
500G	235	60	1	4
600G	282	72	1	5

Grapes

	CALORIES	CARBS	FAT	PROTEIN
5G	4	1	0	0
10G	7	2	0	0

167

20G	14	4	0	0
25G	18	5	0	0
30G	21	6	0	0
40G	28	8	0	0
50G	35	9	0	0
60G	42	11	0	0
70G	49	13	0	0
75G	52	14	0	0
80G	56	15	0	0
90G	63	17	0	0
100G	69	18	0	0
125G	87	23	0	0
150G	104	27	0	1
175G	121	32	0	1
200G	138	36	0	1
300G	207	54	1	2
400G	276	72	1	2
500G	345	90	1	3
600G	414	108	2	4

Mango

	CALORIES	CARBS	FAT	PROTEIN
5G	3	1	0	0
10G	6	2	0	0
20G	12	3	0	0
25G	15	4	0	0
30G	18	5	0	0
40G	24	6	0	0
50G	30	8	0	0
60G	36	9	0	0
70G	42	11	0	0
75G	45	12	0	0
80G	48	12	0	0
90G	54	14	0	0
100G	60	15	0	0
125G	75	19	1	1
150G	90	23	1	1

175G	105	27	1	1
200G	120	30	1	1
300G	180	45	2	2
400G	240	60	2	3
500G	300	75	2	4
600G	360	90	2	4

Watermelon

	CALORIES	CARBS	FAT	PROTEIN
5G	2	1	0	0
10G	3	1	0	0
20G	6	2	0	0
25G	8	2	0	0
30G	9	3	0	0
40G	12	4	0	0
50G	15	4	0	0
60G	18	5	0	0
70G	21	5	0	0
75G	23	6	0	0
80G	24	7	0	0
90G	27	7	0	0
100G	30	8	0	0
125G	38	10	0	0
150G	45	12	0	0
175G	53	14	0	1
200G	60	16	0	1
300G	90	23	0	1
400G	120	31	0	1
500G	150	38	0	3
600G	180	46	0	3

Apricot

	CALORIES	CARBS	FAT	PROTEIN
5G	3	1	0	0
10G	5	2	0	0
20G	10	3	0	0

169

	CALORIES	CARBS	FAT	PROTEIN
25G	12	3	0	0
30G	15	4	0	0
40G	20	5	0	0
50G	24	6	0	0
60G	29	7	0	0
70G	34	8	0	0
75G	36	9	0	1
80G	39	9	0	1
90G	44	10	0	1
100G	48	11	0	1
125G	60	14	0	1
150G	72	17	0	2
175G	84	20	0	2
200G	96	22	0	2
300G	144	33	0	4
400G	192	44	0	5
500G	240	55	0	7
600G	288	66	0	8

Persimmon

	CALORIES	CARBS	FAT	PROTEIN
5G	7	2	0	0
10G	13	4	0	0
20G	26	7	0	0
25G	32	9	0	0
30G	39	11	0	0
40G	51	14	0	0
50G	64	17	0	0
60G	77	21	0	0
70G	89	24	0	0
75G	96	26	0	0
80G	102	28	0	0
90G	115	31	0	0
100G	127	34	0	0
125G	159	43	1	0
150G	191	51	1	1
175G	223	60	1	1

200G	254	68	1	1
300G	381	102	2	2
400G	508	136	2	3
500G	635	170	2	4
600G	762	204	3	4

Passion fruit

	CALORIES	CARBS	FAT	PROTEIN
5G	5	2	0	0
10G	10	3	0	0
20G	20	5	0	0
25G	25	6	0	0
30G	30	7	0	0
40G	39	10	0	0
50G	49	12	0	1
60G	59	14	0	1
70G	68	17	0	1
75G	73	18	1	1
80G	78	19	1	1
90G	88	21	1	1
100G	97	23	1	2
125G	122	29	1	2
150G	146	35	2	3
175G	170	41	2	3
200G	194	46	2	4
300G	291	69	2	7
400G	388	92	3	8
500G	485	115	4	11
600G	582	138	5	13

Kiwi

	CALORIES	CARBS	FAT	PROTEIN
5G	4	1	0	0
10G	7	2	0	0

	CALORIES	CARBS	FAT	PROTEIN
20G	13	3	0	0
25G	16	4	0	0
30G	19	5	0	0
40G	25	6	0	0
50G	31	8	0	0
60G	37	9	0	0
70G	43	11	0	0
75G	46	12	0	0
80G	49	12	0	0
90G	55	14	0	0
100G	61	15	1	1
125G	77	19	1	1
150G	92	23	1	1
175G	107	27	1	1
200G	122	30	1	2
300G	183	45	2	3
400G	244	60	2	4
500G	305	75	3	5
600G	366	90	3	6

Pineapple

	CALORIES	CARBS	FAT	PROTEIN
5G	3	1	0	0
10G	5	2	0	0
20G	10	3	0	0
25G	13	4	0	0
30G	15	4	0	0
40G	20	6	0	0
50G	25	7	0	0
60G	30	8	0	0
70G	35	10	0	0
75G	38	10	0	0
80G	40	11	0	0
90G	45	12	0	0
100G	50	13	0	0
125G	63	17	0	0
150G	75	20	0	0

175G	88	23	0	0
200G	100	26	0	1
300G	150	39	0	1
400G	200	52	0	2
500G	250	65	1	2
600G	300	78	1	3

I'll leave you some space to add your favourite fruits/mixes.

TIP: The easiest way is if you stick to 1 type of fruit per day. You can of course mix them, just make sure you calculate it correctly. Add up your daily fruit allowance and leave most (or all) of it for later. This way, if you need to correct calories or carbs from your previous meals, it's easier. For my breakfast I only use about 20-25g fruit and keep the rest for later.

My favourite fruits

Description	Weight/ amount	Calories	Carbs	Fat	Protein

Description	Weight/amount	Calories	Carbs	Fat	Protein

Treats

This is the best part ☺.

If you were good with your previous macros, you can have some treats. Make sure it fits within your daily calories and macros! If not, then no treats for you ☹

Frozen yoghurt

	CALORIES	CARBS	FAT	PROTEIN
25G	35	3	1	0
50G	69	6	1	1
75G	103	9	2	2
100G	137	12	2	3
125G	172	15	2	4
150G	206	18	3	5

Halo Top protein ice cream

	CALORIES	CARBS	FAT	PROTEIN
25G	19	3	1	0
50G	38	6	2	1
75G	57	9	2	2
100G	76	12	3	3
125G	95	15	3	4
150G	114	18	4	5

Low calories Ben and Jerry's ice cream

	CALORIES	CARBS	FAT	PROTEIN
25G	31	5	2	0
50G	62	9	3	1
75G	93	13	4	1
100G	124	17	5	2
125G	155	22	6	2
150G	186	26	7	3

Popcorn

	CALORIES	CARBS	FAT	PROTEIN
1 SERVING	158	20	8	1
2 SERVINGS	316	40	16	2
3 SERVINGS	474	60	24	3

*Serving size: 30g

Oreo

	CALORIES	CARBS	FAT	PROTEIN
1 SERVING	70	10	4	0
2 SERVINGS	140	20	7	1
3 SERVINGS	210	29	10	1
4 SERVINGS	280	39	13	2

*Serving size: 1 cookie

Bounty

	CALORIES	CARBS	FAT	PROTEIN
1 SERVING	139	17	8	1
2 SERVINGS	278	34	15	2

*Serving size: half bar

Kinder – small bar

	CALORIES	CARBS	FAT	PROTEIN
1 SERVING	71	7	5	1
2 SERVINGS	142	14	9	2
3 SERVINGS	213	21	14	3

*Serving size: 1 bar

Reese's butter cup

	CALORIES	CARBS	FAT	PROTEIN
1 SERVING	87	9	5	1
2 SERVINGS	174	18	10	3
3 SERVINGS	261	27	15	5

*Serving size: 1 piece

Jaffa cake

	CALORIES	CARBS	FAT	PROTEIN
1 SERVING	45	9	1	0
2 SERVINGS	90	17	2	1
3 SERVINGS	135	26	3	1
4 SERVINGS	180	34	4	2

*Serving size: 1 cake

Raffaello

	CALORIES	CARBS	FAT	PROTEIN
1 SERVING	63	4	5	1
2 SERVINGS	126	8	10	2
3 SERVINGS	189	12	15	3

*Serving size: 1 piece

Ferrero Rocher

	CALORIES	CARBS	FAT	PROTEIN
1 SERVING	73	6	6	1
2 SERVINGS	146	11	11	2
3 SERVINGS	219	16	16	3

*Serving size: 1 piece

TIP: I left you some space on the next page, so you can add your favourite treats. If possible, add different amounts of each of them, eg. 1 piece, 2 pieces or 50g, 100g. This way if you can not eat 2 pieces or 100g, you might still be able to have 1 piece or 50g.

My favourite treats

Description	Weight/ amount	Calories	Carbs	Fat	Protein

How to calculate macros from the nutrition label?

I will leave some space for you here, so that you can add your own food and/or brand that   you use.

1. Find the nutrition info of your food. It is either on the packaging or you can search for it online.
2. Find the column that shows nutrition per 100g.
3. Add the name of your food/brand to this table and fill in the nutrition info for 100g (highlighted column).
4. Based on the 100g numbers, calculate macros for other weights.

This is what you need to enter on your calculator
If you want to calculate 10g, you need to multiply your 100g amount with 0.1.
For 20g, it's 0.2. And so on.

10g	x 0.1
20g	x 0.2
25g	x 0.25
30g	x 0.3
40g	x 0.4
50g	x 0.5
60g	x 0.6
70g	x 0.7
80g	x 0.8
90g	x 0.9
100g	x 1 (Find nutrition info on the package.)
110g	x 1.1
120g	x 1.2
200g	x 2
250g	x 2.5
470g	x 4.7

Eg.: If your food shows that 100g is 351 Calories, 83.7C, 0.5F, 1.1P, then 25g of this food will be:

351 x 0.25 = 87.75Cal (I round it up and write 88Cal)
83.7 x 0.25 = 20.925C (so let's say 21C)
0.5 x 0.25 = 0.125 (so basically 0F)
1.1 x 0.25 = 0.275 (so again, it's like 0P)

If it's about calories, carbs and fat, I round it up.
If it's about protein, I round it down.
Eg.: 37.27 Cal, 22.238C, 2.12F, 6.4P
will be: 38Cal, 23C, 3F, 6P
It's easier to work with.

My favourite brands

Description	Weight/ amount	Calories	Carbs	Fat	Protein

Description	Weight/ amount	Calories	Carbs	Fat	Protein

Get organised!

Being organised plays a vital role in succeeding things in our everyday lives. This is certainly the case if you want to stick to your meal plan. You need to know what food and ingredients to buy and how much of it and when/how much to cook. It doesn't matter if you shop once a week and you cook for the whole week in advance or if you shop three times a week and you cook every second or third day, you need to plan time to do it all.

To help you with this, you will find 4 planners below:

1. A list of food and ingredients you like the most and are likely to consume often.
2. A daily meal planner.
3. A weekly meal planner.
4. Emergency shopping list.

My favourite food

This page will include the food you will consume the most of with the amount of weight that fits your meal plan. We are doing this, so you do not have to scroll up and down to find it amongst the tables.

Description	Weight/ amount	Calories	Carbs	Fat	Protein

Description	Weight/ amount	Calories	Carbs	Fat	Protein

Daily meal planner

Breakfast – _____ Cal, _____ C, _____ F, _____ P.

Description	Weight/ amount	Calories	Carbs	Fat	Protein

Lunch/Dinner – _____ Cal, _____ C, _____ F, _____ P.

Description	Weight/ amount	Calories	Carbs	Fat	Protein

Snack – _____ Cal, _____ C, _____ F, _____ P.

Description	Weight/ amount	Calories	Carbs	Fat	Protein

Daily total: _____ Cal, _____ C, _____ F, _____ P.

189

Daily meal planner

Breakfast – _____ Cal, _____ C, _____ F, _____ P.

Description	Weight/ amount	Calories	Carbs	Fat	Protein

Lunch/Dinner – _____ Cal, _____ C, _____ F, _____ P.

Description	Weight/ amount	Calories	Carbs	Fat	Protein

Snack – _____ Cal, _____ C, _____ F, _____ P.

Description	Weight/ amount	Calories	Carbs	Fat	Protein

Daily total: _____ Cal, _____ C, _____ F, _____ P.

Daily meal planner

Breakfast – _____ Cal, _____ C, _____ F, _____ P.

Description	Weight/ amount	Calories	Carbs	Fat	Protein

Lunch/Dinner – _____ Cal, _____ C, _____ F, _____ P.

Description	Weight/ amount	Calories	Carbs	Fat	Protein

Snack – _____ Cal, _____ C, _____ F, _____ P.

Description	Weight/ amount	Calories	Carbs	Fat	Protein

Daily total: _____ Cal, _____ C, _____ F, _____ P.

193

Daily meal planner

Breakfast – _____ Cal, _____ C, _____ F, _____ P.

Description	Weight/ amount	Calories	Carbs	Fat	Protein

Lunch/Dinner – _____ Cal, _____ C, _____ F, _____ P.

Description	Weight/ amount	Calories	Carbs	Fat	Protein

Snack – _____ Cal, _____ C, _____ F, _____ P.

Description	Weight/ amount	Calories	Carbs	Fat	Protein

Daily total: _____ Cal, _____ C, _____ F, _____ P.

195

Daily meal planner

Breakfast – _____ Cal, _____ C, _____ F, _____ P.

Description	Weight/ amount	Calories	Carbs	Fat	Protein

Lunch/Dinner – _____ Cal, _____ C, _____ F, _____ P.

Description	Weight/ amount	Calories	Carbs	Fat	Protein

Snack – _____ Cal, _____ C, _____ F, _____ P.

Description	Weight/ amount	Calories	Carbs	Fat	Protein

Daily total: _____ Cal, _____ C, _____ F, _____ P.

197

Daily meal planner

Breakfast – _____ Cal, _____ C, _____ F, _____ P.

Description	Weight/ amount	Calories	Carbs	Fat	Protein

Lunch/Dinner – _____ Cal, _____ C, _____ F, _____ P.

Description	Weight/ amount	Calories	Carbs	Fat	Protein

Snack – _____ Cal, _____ C, _____ F, _____ P.

Description	Weight/ amount	Calories	Carbs	Fat	Protein

Daily total: _____ Cal, _____ C, _____ F, _____ P.

199

Daily meal planner

Breakfast – _____ Cal, _____ C, _____ F, _____ P.

Description	Weight/ amount	Calories	Carbs	Fat	Protein

Lunch/Dinner – _____ Cal, _____ C, _____ F, _____ P.

Description	Weight/ amount	Calories	Carbs	Fat	Protein

Snack – _____ Cal, _____ C, _____ F, _____ P.

Description	Weight/amount	Calories	Carbs	Fat	Protein

Daily total: _____ Cal, _____ C, _____ F, _____ P.

Daily meal planner

Breakfast – _____ Cal, _____ C, _____ F, _____ P.

Description	Weight/ amount	Calories	Carbs	Fat	Protein

Lunch/Dinner – _____ Cal, _____ C, _____ F, _____ P.

Description	Weight/ amount	Calories	Carbs	Fat	Protein

Snack – _____ Cal, _____ C, _____ F, _____ P.

Description	Weight/ amount	Calories	Carbs	Fat	Protein

Daily total: _____ Cal, _____ C, _____ F, _____ P.

Daily meal planner

Breakfast – _____ Cal, _____ C, _____ F, _____ P.

Description	Weight/ amount	Calories	Carbs	Fat	Protein

Lunch/Dinner – _____ Cal, _____ C, _____ F, _____ P.

Description	Weight/ amount	Calories	Carbs	Fat	Protein

Snack – _____ Cal, _____ C, _____ F, _____ P.

Description	Weight/ amount	Calories	Carbs	Fat	Protein

Daily total: _____ Cal, _____ C, _____ F, _____ P.

Daily meal planner

Breakfast – _____ Cal, _____ C, _____ F, _____ P.

Description	Weight/ amount	Calories	Carbs	Fat	Protein

Lunch/Dinner – _____ Cal, _____ C, _____ F, _____ P.

Description	Weight/ amount	Calories	Carbs	Fat	Protein

Snack – _____ Cal, _____ C, _____ F, _____ P.

Description	Weight/ amount	Calories	Carbs	Fat	Protein

Daily total: _____ Cal, _____ C, _____ F, _____ P.

Weekly meal planner

It can massively help you if you plan your meals for the next week. Based on this you can easily put your shopping list together.

From _____ to _____

	Mon	Tue	Wed	Thu	Fri
Breakfast					
Lunch					
Dinner					
Snack					

Notes:

Weekly meal planner

From _____ to _____

	Mon	Tue	Wed	Thu	Fri
Breakfast					
Lunch					
Dinner					
Snack					

Notes:

209

Weekly meal planner

From _____ to _____

	Mon	Tue	Wed	Thu	Fri
Breakfast					
Lunch					
Dinner					
Snack					

Notes:

Weekly meal planner

From _____ to _____

	Mon	Tue	Wed	Thu	Fri
Breakfast					
Lunch					
Dinner					
Snack					

Notes:

Weekly meal planner

From _____ to _____

	Mon	Tue	Wed	Thu	Fri
Breakfast					
Lunch					
Dinner					
Snack					

Notes:

Weekly meal planner

From _____ to _____

	Mon	Tue	Wed	Thu	Fri
Breakfast					
Lunch					
Dinner					
Snack					

Notes:

Weekly meal planner

From _____ to _____

	Mon	Tue	Wed	Thu	Fri
Breakfast					
Lunch					
Dinner					
Snack					

Notes:

Weekly meal planner

From _____ to _____

	Mon	Tue	Wed	Thu	Fri
Breakfast					
Lunch					
Dinner					
Snack					

Notes:

215

Weekly meal planner

From _____ to _____

	Mon	Tue	Wed	Thu	Fri
Breakfast					
Lunch					
Dinner					
Snack					

Notes:

Weekly meal planner

From _____ to _____

	Mon	Tue	Wed	Thu	Fri
Breakfast					
Lunch					
Dinner					
Snack					

Notes:

217

'Must have at home' list

It's good to stick with the food that is working. I have an "emergency – must have" list that contains all the food I consume on a daily basis and what I do not want to run out of. I therefore keep a good amount of stock.

This is my list and you can create yours too.

- Chicken breast
- Lean beef
- Minced beef
- Rice
- Unsweetened almond milk
- Protein and other supplements
- Stevia
- Peanut butter
- Veg
- Fruit
- Low fat, protein ice cream
- 2 varieties of treats
- Eggs
- Bottled egg white
- Oats
- Chia seeds
- Nuts
- Extra virgin cold pressed coconut oil

My 'must have at home' list

(blank lined list)

Healthy food swap

Here is a chart about what healthy ingredients or methods you can use instead of what you normally use.

NORMALLY	HEALTHY VERSION
WHOLE EGG	Bottled egg white
YOGHURT	0% fat yoghurt
QUARK	Low-fat, high-protein quark
SOFT DRINK	Sugar-free soft drink
MILK	Unsweetened almond milk
COFFEE SYRUP	Sugar-free syrup
SUGAR	Stevia
BUTTER FOR BAKING	Fat-free yoghurt or unsweetened apple sauce or mashed banana or avocado puree or chia seeds
FLOUR FOR BAKING	Instant oat + Protein mix Almond flour + instant oat + protein mix
NOODLES	Konjac noodles
OIL	Extra virgin cold pressed coconut oil
SAUCES	Skinny sauces
COTTAGE CHEESE	Low-fat cottage cheese
BUTTERING THE BAKING TRAY	Baking paper
OIL FOR FRYING EGGS	Non-stick pan
DEEP FRIED	Air fried
SOUR CREAM	Fat-free Greek style yoghurt
SUGAR FOR BAKING	Skinny vanilla extract
PANCAKE MIX	Protein pancake mix
ICE CREAM	Frozen yoghurt, low-fat protein ice cream
CHOCOLATE	Protein bar
NOODLES	Zucchini noodles
TORTILLA WRAP	Low-carb tortilla wrap
SWEETS	Fruit bowl with sugar-free syrup or sweetener (or as it is), sugar-free jelly

I hope you learnt some new things and that this book will make your life easier and save you a lot of time when prepping your meals ☺.

It definitely helped me, I use the very same book. It is all about practice, and I promise it will get easier. Remember, if you calculated something and it works, write it down so you can use it again and again!

If you find any genuine mistakes, I would really appreciate it if you could take the time to let me know on **tiabonn@hotmail.com** so I can rectify it.

If you have any feedback that could make this book better, more useful or more efficient, then please do not hesitate to drop me an email. **tiabonn@hotmail.com**

If you would like to follow me for more tips and meal ideas then you can do so on **Instagram @tia.bonn**
You can also check out my website: tiabonn.com

I would like to thank my friend Alan J Jones for editing my book and translating it from 'Timglish' to 'English'. My lovely cousin Andrea for finding mistakes and last but not least, my dear Brother, Tomi (@tatu_tomi) for doing the graphic design for my cover.

I wish you all the best with your lifestyle change and fitness journey.

xxx

Printed in Great Britain
by Amazon

77452462R00132